ANNALS *of* THE NEW YORK ACADEMY OF SCIENCES

EDITOR-IN-CHIEF
Douglas Braaten

ASSOCIATE EDITOR
Rebecca E. Cooney

PROJECT MANAGER
Steven E. Bohall

EDITORIAL ADMINISTRATOR
Daniel J. Becker

Artwork and design by Ash Ayman Shairzay

The New York Academy of Sciences
7 World Trade Center
250 Greenwich Street, 40th Floor
New York, NY 10007-2157

annals@nyas.org
www.nyas.org/annals

T0337882

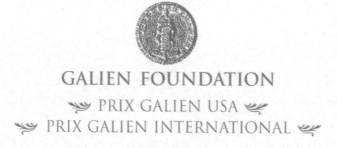

GALIEN FOUNDATION
PRIX GALIEN USA
PRIX GALIEN INTERNATIONAL

ANNALS *of* THE NEW YORK ACADEMY OF SCIENCES

VOLUME
1263

ISSUE

Pharmaceutical Science to Improve the Human Condition: Prix Galien 2011
WINNERS AND FINALIST CANDIDATE OF THE PRIX GALIEN USA AWARDS 2011

TABLE OF CONTENTS

ANNALS OF THE NEW YORK ACADEMY OF SCIENCES

Issue: *Pharmaceutical Science to Improve the Human Condition: Prix Galien 2011*

Development of the IL-12/23 antagonist ustekinumab in psoriasis: past, present, and future perspectives – an update

Newman Yeilding,[1] Philippe Szapary,[1] Carrie Brodmerkel,[1] Jacqueline Benson,[1] Michael Plotnick,[2] Honghui Zhou,[1] Kavitha Goyal,[1] Brad Schenkel,[2] Jill Giles-Komar,[1] Mary Ann Mascelli,[3] and Cynthia Guzzo[1]

[1]Janssen Research & Development, LLC, Spring House, Pennsylvania. [2]Janssen Global Services, LLC, Horsham, Pennsylvania. [3]Biopharmaceutical Consultant, LLC, Ambler, Pennsylvania

Address for correspondence: Newman Yeilding, M.D., Janssen Research & Development, LLC, 1400 McKean Road, Spring House, PA 19477. nyeildin@its.jnj.com

Since the original publication of the article "Development of the IL-12/23 antagonist ustekinumab in psoriasis: Past, present and future perspectives" in March 2011 (see Appendix),[1] there have been several new publications and developments of note. A number of new reports from the ustekinumab psoriasis clinical development program have been published. The analysis of efficacy and safety in the PHOENIX 1 long-term extension demonstrated that continuous stable maintenance dosing of ustekinumab was generally well tolerated and sustained durable efficacy through up to three years of treatment.[2] Pooled safety data from the phase 2 and phase 3 global trials showed that the safety profile of long-term continuous ustekinumab treatment through up to three years[3,4] and four years[5] of follow-up was favorable and comparable to what has been reported previously in the shorter-term ustekinumab psoriasis studies.[6–8] This represents the greatest exposure and longest follow-up of psoriasis patients treated with a biologic published to date. Additional phase 3 trials in Asian populations demonstrated similar high levels of efficacy and favorable safety profiles in Japanese,[9,10] Korean,[11,12] and Taiwanese[11,12] patients as those observed in trials conducted in mostly White populations in North America and Europe.[6–8] These data support the positive benefit:risk profile and consistency of response to ustekinumab over years of usage, and in multiple ethnic groups. Results from up to five years of treatment with ustekinumab in the long-term extensions of the phase 3 trials, and the efficacy, safety, and effect on quality of life in Chinese patients will be available in 2012. In addition to clinical trials of ustekinumab for the treatment of psoriasis, 24-week data from one phase 3 study of ustekinumab for the treatment of psoriatic arthritis has recently been presented[13] and another study is ongoing. A Phase 2b trial in Crohn's disease has also been presented,[14] and three phase 3 studies in Crohn's disease are currently in progress.

Keywords: ustekinumab; psoriasis; human monoclonal antibody; interleukin (IL)-12/23; efficacy; safety; psoriatic arthritis; Crohn's disease

Acknowledgments

The authors wish to thank Dr. Kristin Ruley Sharples of Janssen Biotech, Inc. for her writing support.

Conflicts of interest

The authors are employed by Janssen Research & Development, LLC.

References

1. Yeilding, N., P. Szapary, C. Brodmerkel, *et al.* 2011. Development of the IL-12/23 antagonist ustekinumab in psoriasis: past, present, and future perspectives. *Ann. N.Y. Acad. Sci.* **1222:** 30–39.
2. Kimball, A.B., K.B. Gordon, S. Fakharzadeh, *et al.* 2012. Long-term efficacy of ustekinumab in patients with moderate-to-severe psoriasis: results from the PHOENIX 1 trial through up to 3 years. *Br. J. Dermatol.* **166:** 961–872.

3. Lebwohl, M., C. Leonardi, C.E. Griffiths, *et al.* 2012. Long-term safety experience of ustekinumab in patients with moderate-to-severe psoriasis (part I of II): results from analyses of general safety parameters from pooled Phase 2 and 3 clinical trials. *J. Am. Acad. Dermatol.* **66:** 731–741.

4. Gordon, K. B., K.A. Papp, R.G. Langley, *et al.* 2012. Long-term safety experience of ustekinumab in patients with moderate to severe psoriasis (part II of II): results from analyses of infections and malignancy from pooled phase II and III clinical trials. *J. Am. Acad. Dermatol.* **66:** 742–751.

5. Reich, K., K.A. Papp, C.E.M. Griffiths, *et al.* 2012. An update on the long-term safety experience of ustekinumab: results from the psoriasis clinical development program with up to four years of follow-up. *J. Drugs Dermatol.* **11:** 300–312.

6. Leonardi, C.L., A.B. Kimball, K.A. Papp, *et al.* 2008. Efficacy and safety of ustekinumab, a human interleukin-12/23 monoclonal antibody, in patients with psoriasis: 76-week results from a randomised, double-blind, placebo-controlled trial (PHOENIX 1). *Lancet* **371:** 1665–1674.

7. Papp, K.A., R.G. Langley, M. Lebwohl, *et al.* 2008. Efficacy and safety of ustekinumab, a human interleukin-12/23 monoclonal antibody, in patients with psoriasis: 52-week results from a randomised, double-blind, placebo-controlled trial (PHOENIX 2). *Lancet* **371:** 1675–1684.

8. Griffiths, C.E., B.E. Strober, P. van de Kerkof, *et al.* 2010. Comparison of ustekinumab and etanercept for moderate-to-severe psoriasis. *N. Engl. J. Med.* **362:** 118–128.

9. Igarashi, A., T. Kato, M. Kato, *et al.*, THE JAPANESE USTEKINUMAB STUDY GROUP. 2012. Efficacy and safety of ustekinumab in Japanese patients with moderate-to-severe plaque-type psoriasis: Long-term results from a phase 2/3 clinical trial. *J. Dermatol.* **39:** 242–252.

10. Nakagawa, H., B. Schenkel, M. Kato, *et al.* 2012. Impact of ustekinumab on health-related quality of life in Japanese patients with moderate-to-severe plaque psoriasis: results from a randomized, double-blind, placebo-controlled Phase 2/3 trial. *J. Dermatol.* Mar 13. [Epub ahead of print].

11. Tsai, T.F., J.C. Ho, M. Song, *et al.*, PEARL Investigators. 2011. Efficacy and safety of ustekinumab for the treatment of moderate-to-severe psoriasis: a phase III, randomized, placebo-controlled trial in Taiwanese and Korean patients (PEARL). *J. Dermatol. Sci.* **63:** 154–163.

12. Tsai, T.F., M. Song, Y-K. Shen, *et al.* 2012. Ustekinumab improves health-related quality of life in Korean and Taiwanese patients with moderate-to-severe psoriasis: Results from the PEARL trial. *J. Drugs Dermatol.* in press.

13. McInnes, I., A. Kavanaugh, A. Gottlieb, *et al.* Ustekinumab in patients with active psoriatic arthritis: results of the phase 3, multicenter, double-blind, placebo-controlled PSUMMIT I study. Abstract to be presented at: The European League Against Rheumatism (EULAR); June 8, 2012; Berlin, Germany. Oral Presentation OP0158.

14. Sandborn, W.J., C. Gasink, L-L. Gao, *et al.* A multicenter, randomized, double-blind, placebo-controlled phase 2b study of ustekinumab, a human monoclonal antibody to IL-12/23p40, in patients with moderately to severely active Crohn's disease: results through week 22 from the CERTIFI Trial. Abstract presented at: Digestive Disease Week (DDW); May 19–22, 2012; San Diego, CA, USA. Abstract 1031129.

Appendix

Yeilding, N., Szapary, P., Brodmerkel, C., Benson, J., Plotnick, M., Zhou, H., Goyal, K., Schenkel, B., Giles-Komar, J., Mascelli, M. A. and Guzzo, C. 2011. Development of the IL-12/23 antagonist ustekinumab in psoriasis: past, present, and future perspectives. *Ann. N.Y. Acad. Sci.* **1222:** 30–39. doi: 10.1111/j.1749-6632.2011.05963.x

Ann. N.Y. Acad. Sci. ISSN 0077-8923

ANNALS OF THE NEW YORK ACADEMY OF SCIENCES
Issue: *Pharmaceutical Science to Improve the Human Condition: Prix Galien 2010*

Development of the IL-12/23 antagonist ustekinumab in psoriasis: past, present, and future perspectives

Newman Yeilding,[1] Philippe Szapary,[1] Carrie Brodmerkel,[1] Jacqueline Benson,[1] Michael Plotnick,[2] Honghui Zhou,[1] Kavitha Goyal,[1] Brad Schenkel,[2] Jill Giles-Komar,[1] Mary Ann Mascelli,[3] and Cynthia Guzzo[1]

[1]Centocor Research and Development, Inc., Malvern, Pennsylvania. [2]Janssen Global Services, LLC, Horsham, Pennsylvania. [3]Biopharmaceutical Consultant, LLC, Ambler, Pennsylvania

Address for correspondence: Newman Yeilding, Centocor Research and Development, Inc., 965 Chesterbrook Boulevard, Wayne, PA 19087. nyeildin@its.jnj.com

The development of ustekinumab as a first-in-class anti-interleukin (IL) 12/23p40 therapeutic agent for psoriasis represents an important example of modern and rational drug design and development. Psoriasis is a chronic, systemic, immune-mediated skin disorder with considerable clinical, psychosocial, and economic burden. Ustekinumab is a human monoclonal antibody (mAb) that binds the p40 subunit common to IL-12 and IL-23, key cytokines in psoriasis pathogenesis. The therapeutic mAb was developed using human gamma-1 immunoglobulin (IgG)-expressing transgenic mice, which created a molecule with endogenous IgG_1 biologic properties and low immunogenicity. Ustekinumab was well tolerated in clinical studies and yielded rapid, significant, and sustained efficacy plus improved quality of life/work performance and reduced depression/anxiety. Its pharmacologic properties afford the most convenient dosing regimen among approved biologics, representing a significant advancement in the treatment of moderate to severe psoriasis. Ustekinumab also holds promise for other immune-mediated disorders with significant unmet need.

Keywords: ustekinumab; psoriasis; human monoclonal antibody (mAb); Dermatology Life Quality Index (DLQI); Psoriasis Activity and Severity Index (PASI); Hospital Anxiety and Depression Score (HADS)

Epidemiologic, clinical, and pathologic manifestations of psoriasis

Psoriasis is the most common chronic, immune-mediated skin disorder, affecting approximately 2% of the world's population.[1] Psoriasis is characterized by thickened epidermal layers resulting from excessive keratinocyte (KC) cell proliferation. The majority of sufferers are afflicted with psoriasis for most of their lives. Symptoms typically present between the ages of 15 and 35, with the majority of individuals diagnosed before the age of 40.[2]

Plaque psoriasis is the most common form, affecting approximately 85–90% of individuals with the condition. The disease manifests as raised, well-demarcated, erythematous, and frequently pruritic/painful plaques with silvery scales.[3,4] Plaques are commonly seen on the elbows, knees, lower back, and umbilical area, although many patients have plaques on cosmetically sensitive areas and/or regions that cause substantial discomfort, such as the scalp, face, hands, feet, and genitalia. Approximately 25% of individuals with psoriasis develop moderate to severe disease with widely disseminated lesions.[3,4]

Psoriasis is also associated with multiple comorbidities, including psoriatic arthritis (PsA), depression, cardiovascular disease, hypertension, obesity, diabetes, metabolic syndrome, and Crohn's disease.[5] Recently, the National Psoriasis Foundation issued a clinical consensus on comorbidities observed in psoriasis patients and provided clinicians with recommendations for disease screening.[6]

In addition to the impact of significant comorbidities, psoriasis also imposes physical and psychosocial burdens that extend beyond the physical

doi: 10.1111/j.1749-6632.2011.05963.x

dermatological symptoms. When lesions are located in sensitive areas, psoriasis can interfere with everyday activities. Psoriasis negatively impacts familial and spousal relationships, as well as other social and work relationships.[7,8] Psoriasis is associated with a higher incidence of depression and increased suicidal tendencies, particularly in young adults (18 to 34 years old), compared with the broader population.[9] Finally, individuals with psoriasis generally have reduced levels of employment, job retention, and income.[10]

Psoriasis treatment modalities

Multiple therapeutic options existed for the treatment of moderate to severe psoriasis prior to ustekinumab's development. However, a significant unmet need remained for a safe, highly effective, convenient systemic therapy.[11] Psoralen plus ultraviolet A light therapy, while effective, is inconvenient and is associated with an increased risk of skin malignancies and photodamage. Significant safety concerns and organ toxicity are associated with chronic administration of conventional systemic agents such as methotrexate, cyclosporine, and acitretin, thus limiting their use in long-term psoriasis management. Other biologic agents approved for the treatment of psoriasis have suboptimal and/or diminishing efficacy, inconvenient modes and/or schedules of administration, and associated drug-specific safety concerns (e.g., infections including tuberculosis, malignancies including lymphoma, and demyelinating neurologic disorders). For currently available subcutaneous (s.c.) agents, efficacy is limited in cases of obesity, a comorbidity commonly observed in psoriasis patients. The need for an optimal therapeutic agent was highlighted by the results of patient surveys that revealed general dissatisfaction with available therapies resulting, at least in part, from dissatisfaction with effectiveness or convenience of available treatments.[12,13]

Targeting the underlying pathology of psoriasis: the role of interleukins 12 and 23

Aberrant immune-mediated inflammatory responses are associated with psoriasis pathogenesis, and certain inflammatory cytokines/pathways have been studied as therapeutic targets.[14] In the mid-1990s, analysis of human psoriatic plaque tissue and animal models suggested that both IL-12 and the immune T helper 1 (Th1) effector lineage corre-

lated with psoriasis pathophysiology.[15,16] IL-12 is a heterodimeric protein comprising two disulfide-linked, glycosylated subunits, designated p35 and p40, which is secreted by antigen-presenting cells in response to inflammatory stimuli or infection (Fig. 1A). The IL-12 cytokine activates natural killer (NK) and T cell responses, including CD4$^+$ T cell differentiation toward the Th1 phenotype.[17] Subsequent to ustekinumab generation, a second heterodimeric cytokine containing the identical p40 subunit disulfide-linked with a p19 subunit was reported.[18] This cytokine, named IL-23, has demonstrated activity against NK and T cell populations, including Th17 lineages.[19,20]

Results of numerous studies suggest that IL-12 and IL-23 may play a central role in psoriasis pathogenesis. Polymorphisms of genes that encode either the shared p40 subunit or one of the IL-23 receptor (IL-23R) complex components are linked to psoriasis.[21] An uncommon IL-23R coding variant that confers protection against Crohn's disease has also been shown to confer protection against psoriasis.[22,23] Gene expression levels of IL-12, interferon gamma (IFN-γ), and IL-23 are elevated in psoriasis skin lesions.[24] Indeed, many psoriasis therapies used prior to ustekinumab approval modulate IL-12 and IL-23 levels, a mechanism speculated to contribute to their efficacy.[24,25]

Th1 and Th17 cells contribute to psoriasis pathophysiology by secreting inflammatory cytokines, including IFN-γ, IL-17, and IL-22, that then activate KCs to proliferate and secrete additional inflammatory mediators. Collectively, immune cell infiltration into the skin and the resulting inflammatory processes result in psoriasis skin pathology. The production of IL-12 and IL-23 and their downstream impact on Th1 and Th17 activation, as well as KC activation, are illustrated in Figure 1B. Based on these pathways, a therapeutic agent designed to block IL-12 and IL-23 was also anticipated to block IL-12– and IL-23–mediated Th1 and Th17 cell production of IFN-γ, IL-17, and IL-22, thereby ameliorating KC activation and enabling normalization of skin pathology.

Generation of ustekinumab: a monoclonal antibody with novel therapeutic attributes

Ustekinumab was developed as a monoclonal antibody (mAb) designed to block IL-12. The therapeutic mAb was generated using the human

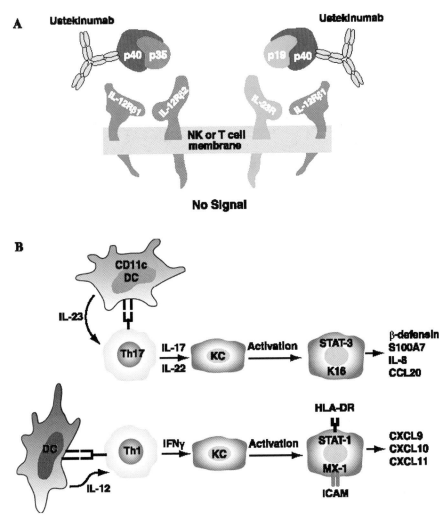

Figure 1. Ustekinumab mechanism of action: the role of T helper (Th) 1/Th17 pathways in the pathophysiology of plaque psoriasis. (A) Illustration of ustekinumab, IL-12, and IL-23, and their respective receptors. Ustekinumab binds to the p40 subunit of IL-12 and IL-23, and prevents the cytokines' interaction with the cell surface IL-12 receptor β1 (IL-12Rβ1) and subsequently inhibits IL-12 and IL-23–mediated cell signaling, activation, and cytokine production. Adapted from Dillon,[47] Figure 1. (B) Proposed roles of Th1 and Th17 cells in keratinocyte (KC) activation and proliferation. Activated dendritic cells (DCs) produce IL-23, which supports Th17 cell survival/proliferation and induces production of IL-17 and IL-22. DC and Th17 cell products activate KCs and promote release of innate immunity molecules such as β-defensin, S100 calcium-binding protein A7 (S100A7), IL-8, and chemokine (C-C motif) ligand 20 (CCL20). Concurrently, Th1 cells produce IFN-γ, which induces KCs to upregulate major histocompatibility complex (MHC) class II molecule human leukocyte antigen (HLA-DR) and integrins such as intracellular adhesion molecule (ICAM), and release cytokines including C-X-C motif (CXCL) 9, CXCL10, and CXCL11. Th1 and Th17 cells may suppress each other's development, but IFN-γ can also act synergistically with IL-17 to increase expression and IL-8 release from KCs.[48] Adapted from Zaba,[49] Figure 6.

immunoglobulin (Ig)–expressing transgenic mice developed by Medarex (formally GenPharm, Princeton, NJ) that contain human Ig heavy- and light-chain variable- and constant-region genes.[26] A major advantage of transgenic technology is that the mice are capable of producing human antibodies following antigen challenge employing the same hybridoma technology used to generate murine mAbs (Fig. 2). The human antibodies generated by transgenic technology were anticipated to have half-lives comparable to endogenous gamma-1 Ig (IgG₁) and lower rates of immunogenicity.

Ustekinumab was generated by first immunizing the Medarex mice with human IL-12, followed by

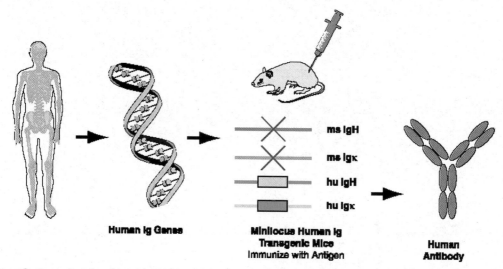

Figure 2. Generation of ustekinumab. Ustekinumab was generated using transgenic mice engineered to express human antibodies. Human heavy-, and light-chain antibody genes were used by Medarex to prepare minilocus human immunoglobulin (IgH) transgenic mice. Upon challenge with antigen, the transgenic mice produce human antibodies. ms = mouse; hu = human.

performance of hybridoma fusions using spleens of mice demonstrating titers for human IL-12. The properties of ustekinumab obviated the need for additional affinity maturation via molecular engineering. Ustekinumab was found to neutralize IL-12 by binding the p40 subunit and thereby preventing IL-12 binding to the IL-12β1 chain of the IL-12R complex. Subsequent to the discovery of IL-23, ustekinumab was found to similarly neutralize IL-23 bioactivity by binding the shared p40 subunit and preventing interaction with the IL-12β1 chain of the IL-23R complex. Molecular analysis further demonstrated that ustekinumab binds to domain 1 of IL-12/23p40 with the expected 2:1 cytokine-to-antibody stoichiometry.[27] The ability of ustekinumab to bind to the p40 subunit of both IL-12 and IL-23 is the basis for dual neutralization of IL-12 and IL-23 biological activity (Fig. 1A).

Ustekinumab psoriasis clinical experience

Promise revealed in early clinical development
Ustekinumab's therapeutic potential was apparent in the early phase 1 trials conducted in patients with moderate to severe psoriasis.[28–30] Results of these phase 1 trials demonstrated an elimination half-life of approximately 3 weeks, consistent with endogenous IgG1. Moreover, ustekinumab was well tolerated and appeared to have low immunogenic potential. Reductions in lesional gene expression of

IL-12p40, IL-23p19, and other inflammatory cytokines were significant as early as 2 weeks post-treatment. Importantly, in some individuals with psoriasis, a single intravenous (i.v.) or s.c. dose of ustekinumab resulted in rapid and marked clinical response that was sustained for 16–24 weeks (photographs of a representative patient are shown in Fig. 3), indicating that ustekinumab has the potential to be a highly effective, yet convenient, psoriasis therapy.

Promise confirmed in late-stage clinical development
Ustekinumab's safety and efficacy were further assessed in three large phase 3 trials involving 2,899 patients with moderate to severe psoriasis. Results of the placebo-controlled PHOENIX 1 and PHOENIX 2 phase 3 trials demonstrated that ustekinumab is highly effective in ameliorating psoriatic plaques, pruritus, and nail psoriasis (photographs of a representative patient are shown in the top of Fig. 4).[31,32] Within 12 weeks of initiating ustekinumab treatment (45 mg/kg or 90 mg/kg at weeks 0 and 4), more than two-thirds of patients experienced ≥75% reduction in the Psoriasis Area and Severity Index (PASI 75) score (bottom of Fig. 4; panel A). Maximum efficacy was achieved at approximately 24 weeks after initiation of therapy, with approximately 75% of ustekinumab-treated patients achieving a PASI 75 response. Similar response patterns

0.1 mg/kg dose group

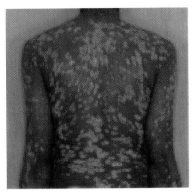
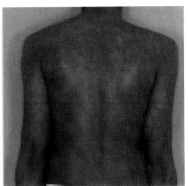

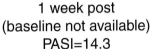

1 week post
(baseline not available)
PASI=14.3

16 weeks post
PASI=0.5

Figure 3. Photographs of a representative patient from the ustekinumab first-in-human, phase 1 study in moderate to severe psoriasis. The patient received a single intravenous (i.v.) administration of the lowest evaluated dose of ustekinumab (0.1 mg/kg). Images were obtained at 1 and 16 weeks following ustekinumab administration. The patient's Psoriasis Activity and Severity Index (PASI) score decreased from 14.3 at 1 week following dosing to 0.5 at week 16. Adapted from Kauffman,[29] Figure 4.

were observed for the proportions of patients with Physician's Global Assessment (PGA) score of 0 or 1, PASI 90 response, and/or PASI 50 response (bottom of Fig. 4; panels B, C, and D, respectively). Because its half-life is consistent with that of endogenous IgG1, ustekinumab is not rapidly cleared from the body, yielding a high level of clinical response sustained with convenient every 12-week maintenance dosing in approximately 80% of responding patients. Clinical response to ustekinumab was associated with serum ustekinumab concentrations that were affected by patient body weight. While efficacy of the 45 and 90 mg doses of ustekinumab was similar in patients weighing ≤100 kg, the 90 mg dose was more effective than the 45 mg dose in patients weighing >100 kg, who represented approximately one-third of the combined PHOENIX 1 and 2 population. Thus, to optimize efficacy in all patients while minimizing unnecessary drug exposure, fixed dose administration of ustekinumab based on body weight is indicated in the treatment of psoriasis such that 45 mg is employed for patients weighing ≤100 and 90 mg is recommended for patients weighing >100 kg.

In the ACCEPT phase 3 trial,[33] ustekinumab's safety and efficacy were compared with those of etanercept, the biologic agent most commonly prescribed for psoriasis. Results of the first ever head-to-head trial of two biologic agents for psoriasis demonstrated the superior efficacy at week 12 of both ustekinumab 45 and 90 mg, when administered at weeks 0 and 4 in patients with moderate to severe psoriasis, versus high-dose etanercept (50 mg) when administered twice weekly for 12 weeks. In addition, nearly one-half of patients who had not responded to etanercept subsequently responded to ustekinumab.

Ustekinumab improves multiple patient-reported outcomes

The robust clinical efficacy observed in ustekinumab-treated patients in the pivotal phase 3 studies translated into improved health-related quality of life (HRQoL). In the PHOENIX 1 and 2 phase 3 trials, the skin disease-specific HRQoL assessment, the Dermatology Life Quality Index (DLQI), revealed significant improvement in patient-reported QoL. The mean baseline DLQI score in both trials was >10, indicating substantial QoL impairment. However, more than 50% of patients reported no impairment of QoL (DLQI score = 0 or 1) after 12 weeks of ustekinumab treatment, compared with only 3.2% of placebo-treated patients.[34,35] Additionally, the mean improvement in DLQI was significantly greater for ustekinumab- versus placebo-treated patients (Fig. 5A). After crossing over to receive ustekinumab at week 12,

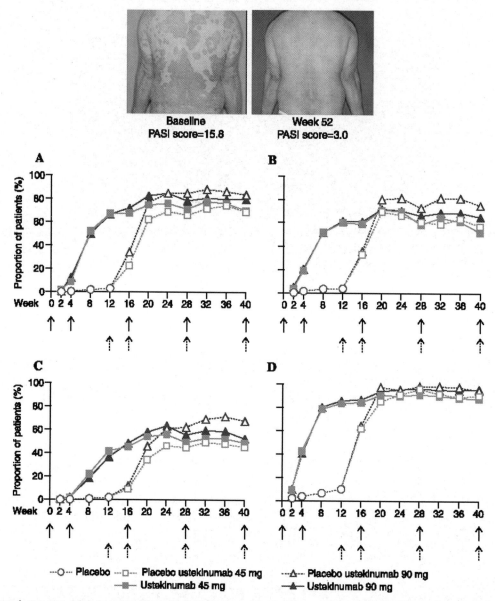

Figure 4. Extent and duration of ustekinumab clinical response. Top: Baseline and post-treatment photographs of a representative patient from the PHOENIX 1 phase 3 study randomized to treatment with ustekinumab 45 mg at weeks 0, 4, 16, 28, and 40. Images were obtained at baseline and week 52. Bottom: Proportions of randomized patients in the PHOENIX 1 phase 3 study who achieved clinical response from baseline through week 40, as assessed by the Psoriasis Area and Severity Index (PASI) 75 response criteria (A); Physician's Global Assessment (PGA) of cleared or minimal (0 or 1) (B); PASI 90 response criteria (C); and PASI 50 response criteria (D). For week 28 PASI 50 nonresponders, data at week 28 were carried forward to weeks 32, 36, and 40. The arrows indicate visits at which ustekinumab was administered to patients randomized to receive ustekinumab at baseline (solid arrows) and to those randomized to receive placebo at weeks 0 and 4, followed by ustekinumab at weeks 12, 16, 28, and 40 (dotted arrows). From Leonardi,[31] Figure 3.

patients initially receiving placebo subsequently achieved improvements in DLQI. Importantly, improvement in patient-reported outcomes was observed as early as week 4 in the trials.

Ustekinumab also improved depression and anxiety symptoms, which are common psoriasis comorbidities, based on analyses of the Hospital Anxiety and Depression Scale (HADS) in the PHOENIX 2

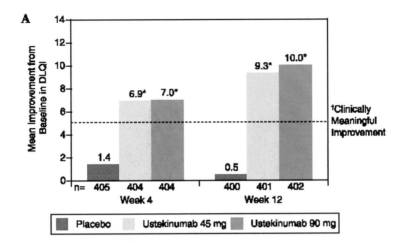

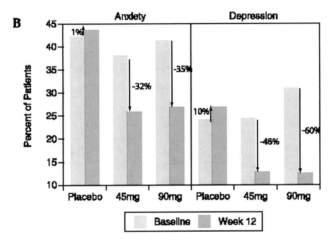

Figure 5. Impact of ustekinumab on patient-reported outcomes. (A) Mean improvement from baseline in Dermatology Life Quality Index (DLQI) scores at weeks 4 and 12 in the phase 3 PHOENIX 1 trial following receipt of study agent at weeks 0 and 4.[31] A ≥5-point change in the DLQI score represents clinically meaningful improvement.[50] (B) Percentage of patients in the PHOENIX 2 phase 3 trial with Hospital Anxiety and Depression Score (HADS) >7 at baseline and week 12 (following dosing at weeks 0 and 4).[34]

trial.[34] Approximately one-third of patients entering the study reported mild-to-severe symptoms of anxiety, and one-quarter of patients reported mild-to-severe symptoms of depression. By week 12, after two ustekinumab doses at weeks 0 and 4, the overall proportions of ustekinumab-treated patients exhibiting symptoms decreased by 34% for anxiety and 55% for depression. In contrast, the proportions of placebo-treated patients with anxiety and depression symptoms at week 12 increased by 1% and 10%, respectively (Fig. 5B).

Ustekinumab treatment also significantly improved other patient-reported outcomes evaluated in the phase 3 trials, including the Itch Visual Analog

Scale, the Medical Outcomes Study 36-item short-form health survey (SF-36), and the Work Limitations Questionnaire (WLQ), evaluating on-the-job limitations such as physical, time management, and productivity impairments. Thus, findings related to patient-reported outcomes indicate that ustekinumab yields significant and meaningful improvement in both the physical and psychosocial comorbidities associated with moderate to severe psoriasis.[34,35]

Tolerability of ustekinumab

Results of the phase 3 psoriasis clinical trials indicated that ustekinumab was generally well tolerated. Rates and types of adverse events (AEs), serious AEs, AEs leading to treatment discontinuation, and laboratory abnormalities were generally comparable among patients receiving placebo, ustekinumab 45 and 90 mg during the 12-week placebo-controlled phases of PHOENIX 1 and 2. Dose-response relationships for safety events were not apparent. Immunogenicity rates were low, with approximately 5% of patients developing anti-ustekinumab antibodies, and drug administration was well tolerated, with approximately 1% of injections having an associated injection site reaction.[31,32]

Blocking IL-12 and/or IL-23 carries theoretical risks of infection and suppression of tumor immune surveillance.[36] For instance, mycobacterial and salmonella infections were reported in individuals congenitally deficient in IL-12p40 or IL-12Rβ1.[37] Rates of serious infections and malignancies in PHOENIX 1 and 2 were low and comparable across treatment groups during the placebo-controlled phases, no apparent increase in the frequency of these AEs was observed through 18 months of treatment, and no mycobacterial or salmonella infections were reported.[31,32] A more complete characterization of ustekinumab safety will require continued vigilance as more patients are treated for extended periods. To achieve this aim, a multifaceted global risk management plan is in place that includes 5 years of long-term follow-up in PHOENIX 1 and 2, a disease-based registry (PSOLAR) comprising 4,000 patients exposed to ustekinumab and 8,000 patients exposed to other biologic and/or oral systemic psoriasis treatments, analyses across several registries and healthcare claims databases, and ongoing pharmacovigilance activities.

Future promise

While initially developed as a treatment for psoriasis, ustekinumab also holds promise for other immune-mediated inflammatory disorders. Animal model, clinical, and translational data have established a strong associative and causal link between dysregulation of the Th1 and/or Th17 pathways and numerous rheumatic (rheumatoid arthritis, PsA),[38] metabolic (type 1 diabetes),[39] gastrointestinal (Crohn's, ulcerative colitis, primary biliary cirrhosis),[40,41] and neurologic (multiple sclerosis

[MS])[42] disorders, as well as the multiorgan granulomatous disease, sarcoidosis.[43]

Early-stage human clinical trials have demonstrated the therapeutic potential of ustekinumab in Crohn's disease[44] and PsA,[45] although a therapeutic benefit was not observed in MS.[46] In a phase 2 PsA study, ustekinumab significantly reduced signs and symptoms of PsA and improved skin lesions after two SC doses. Results of a phase 2 study in patients with moderate to severe Crohn's disease indicated that ustekinumab improved signs and symptoms, and induced clinical response within 4 to 6 weeks of initiating treatment. Ongoing phase 3 trials aim to establish the benefit-risk profile of ustekinumab in PsA. A phase 2 study evaluating the efficacy of ustekinumab in sarcoidosis is also ongoing. In combination, observations to date suggest that ustekinumab has potential not only as a new standard for treating psoriasis, but also as a promising therapeutic agent for other immune-mediated inflammatory diseases in which IL-12 and/or IL-23 play a pathogenic role.

Summary and future perspectives

Ustekinumab is a significant and innovative advancement in the treatment of moderate to severe plaque psoriasis. The agent is one of the first therapeutic mAbs approved for human use that was developed in Medarex transgenic mice, which produce human mAbs for therapeutic applications. The ustekinumab clinical development program is an important example of modern drug development incorporating a strong emphasis on translational medicine, pharmacology, and rational drug design. The molecular, pharmacologic, and clinical attributes of ustekinumab translate into rapid, substantial, and sustained therapeutic benefit for patients with psoriasis. The benefits of ustekinumab extend beyond attenuation of disease, as evidenced by significant improvements of the physical and psychosocial burdens associated with psoriasis, including anxiety and depression. Ustekinumab's less-frequent dosing requirements set a new standard for convenience of psoriasis therapies. Its high degree of efficacy, tolerability, and convenient dose regimen are anticipated to set the standard for future treatment compliance and satisfaction. Additional safety data through 5 years in these pivotal trials, as well as from registries, databases, and pharmacovigilance activities, will further define the ustekinumab safety profile. Emerging research indicates that the Th1/Th17 pathways are involved in a diverse array of immune-mediated disorders. Early-phase clinical trial results suggest that ustekinumab may also prove effective in treating PsA and Crohn's disease, thus expanding the therapeutic landscape for IL12/23p40 inhibitors. Future clinical development will determine the full promise of these agents for immune-mediated inflammatory disorders.

Acknowledgments

The authors want to thank Dr. Mary Whitman for her critical review of the document.

Conflicts of interest

N. Yeilding, C. Brodmerkel, J. Benson, P. Szapary, K. Goyal, J. Giles-Komar, C. Guzzo, and H. Zhou are employees of Centocor Research and Development, Inc. B. Schenkel and M. Plotnick are employees of Janssen Global Services, LLC—all subsidiaries of Johnson & Johnson. M. Mascelli is a paid consultant for Centocor Ortho Biotech Services, LLC. All authors are Johnson & Johnson stockholders.

References

1. Nestle, F.O., D.H. Kaplan & J. Barker. 2009. Psoriasis. *N. Engl. J. Med.* **361:** 496–509.
2. Farber, E.M. & L. Nall. 1998. Natural history and genetics. In *Psoriasis*, 3rd ed., H.H. Roenigk Jr. & Hi Maibach, Eds.: 114–115. Marcel Dekker. New York.
3. Christophers, E. 2001. Psoriasis—epidemiology and clinical spectrum. *Clin. Exp. Dermatol.* **26:** 314–320.
4. Griffiths, C.E. & J.N. Barker. 2007. Pathogenesis and clinical features of psoriasis. *Lancet* **370:** 263–271.
5. Mrowietz, U., J.T. Elder & J. Barker. 2006. The importance of disease associations and concomitant therapy for the long-term management of psoriasis patients. *Arch. Dermatol. Res.* **298:** 309–319.
6. Kimball, A.B., D. Gladman, J.M. Gelfand, *et al.* 2008. National Psoriasis Foundation clinical consensus on psoriasis comorbidities and recommendations for screening. *J. Am. Acad. Dermatol.* **58:** 1031–1042.
7. Eghlileb, A.M., E.E.G. Davies & A.Y. Finlay. 2007. Psoriasis has a major secondary impact on the lives of family members and partners. *Brit. J. Dermatol.* **156:** 1245–1250.
8. Basra, M.K.A. & A.Y. Finlay. 2007. The family impact of skin diseases: the Greater Patient concept. *Brit. J. Dermatol.* **156:** 929–937.
9. Picardi, A., E. Mazzotti & P. Pasquini. 2006. Prevalence and correlates of suicide ideation among patients with skin disease. *J. Am. Acad. Dermatol.* **54:** 420–426.
10. Horn, E.J., K.M. Fox, V. Patel, *et al.* 2007. Association of patient-reported psoriasis severity with income and employment. *J. Am. Acad. Dermatol.* **57:** 963–971.
11. Canadian Psoriasis Guidelines Committee, 2009. Canadian Guidelines for the Management of Plaque Psoriasis.
12. Stern, R.S., T. Nijsten, S.R. Feldman, *et al.* 2004. Psoriasis is common, carries a substantial burden even when not extensive, and is associated with widespread treatment dissatisfaction. *J. Investig. Dermatol. Symp. Proc.* **9:** 136–139.
13. Richards, H.L., D.G. Fortune & C.E.M. Griffiths. 2006. Adherence to treatment in patients with psoriasis. *J.E.A.D.V.* **20:** 370–379.
14. Nickoloff, B.J. & F.O. Nestle. 2004. Recent insights into the immunopathogenesis of psoriasis provide new therapeutic opportunities. *J. Clin. Invest.* **113:** 1664–1675.
15. Hong, K., A. Chu, B.R. Lúdviksson, *et al.* 1999. IL-12, independently of IFN-gamma, plays a crucial role in the pathogenesis of a murine psoriasis-like skin disorder. *J. Immunol.* **162:** 7480–7491.
16. Yawalker, N., S. Karlen, R. Hunger, *et al.* 1998. Expression of interleukin-12 is increased in psoriatic skin. *J. Invest. Dermatol.* **111:** 1053–1057.
17. Trinchieri, G. 2003. Interleukin-12 and the regulation of innate resistance and adaptive immunity. *Nat. Rev. Immunol.* **3:** 133–146.
18. Oppmann, B., R. Lesley, B. Blom, *et al.* 2000. Novel p19 protein engages IL-12p40 to form a cytokine, IL-23, with biological activities similar as well as distinct from IL-12. *Immunity* **13:** 715–725.
19. Aggarwal, S., N. Ghilardi, M-H. Xie, *et al.* 2003. Interleukin-23 promotes a distinct CD4 T cell activation state characterized by the production of interleukin-17. *J. Biol. Chem.* **278:** 1910–1914.
20. Wilson, N.J., K. Boniface, J.R. Chan, *et al.* 2007. Development, cytokine profile and function of human interleukin 17-producing helper T cells. *Nat. Immunol.* **8:** 950–957.
21. Cargill, M., S.J. Schrodi, M. Chang, *et al.* 2007. A large-scale genetic association study confirms *IL12B* and leads to the identification of *IL23R* as psoriasis-risk genes. *Am. J. Hum. Genet.* **80:** 273–290.
22. Duerr, R.H., K.D. Taylor, S.R. Brant, *et al.* 2006. A genome-wide association study identifies *IL23R* as an inflammatory bowel disease gene. *Science* **314:** 1461–1463.
23. Capon, F., P. Di Meglio, J. Szaub, *et al.* 2007. Sequence variants in the genes for the interleukin-23 receptor (IL23R) and its ligand (IL12B) confer protection against psoriasis. *Hum. Genet.* **122:** 201–206.
24. Torti, D.C. & S.R. Feldman. 2007. Interleukin-12, interleukin-23, and psoriasis: current prospects. *J. Am. Acad. Dermatol.* **57:** 1059–1068. Comment and author reply.
25. Zaba, L.C., M. Suárez-Fariñas, J. Fuentes-Duculan, *et al.* 2009. Effective treatment of psoriasis with etanercept is linked to suppression of IL-17 signaling, not immediate response TNF genes. *J. Allergy Clin. Immunol.* **124:** 1022–1030.
26. Fishwild, D.M., S.L. O'Donnell, T. Bengoechea, *et al.* 1996. High-avidity human IgG kappa monoclonal antibodies from a novel strain of minilocus transgenic mice. *Nat. Biotechnol.* **14:** 845–851.
27. Luo, J., S.J. Wu, E.R. Lacy, *et al.* 2010. Structural basis for the dual recognition of IL-12 and IL-23 by ustekinumab. *J. Mol. Biol.* **402:** 797–812.
28. Toichi, E., G. Torres, T.S. McCormick, *et al.* 2006. An anti-IL-12p40 antibody down-regulates type 1 cytokines,

chemokines, and IL-12/IL-23 in psoriasis. *J. Immunol.* **177:** 4917–4926.

29. Kauffman, C.L., N. Aria, E. Toichi, *et al.* 2004. A phase I study evaluating the safety, pharmacokinetics, and clinical response of a human IL-12 antibody in subjects with plaque psoriasis. *J. Invest. Dermatol.* **123:** 1037–1044.

30. Gottlieb, A.B., K.D. Cooper, T.S. McCormick, *et al.* 2007. A phase I, double-blind, placebo-controlled study evaluating single subcutaneous administrations of a human interleukin-12/23 monoclonal antibody in subjects with plaque psoriasis. *Curr. Med. Res. Opin.* **23:** 1081–1092.

31. Leonardi, C.L., A.B. Kimball, K.A. Papp, *et al.* 2008. Efficacy and safety of ustekinumab, a human interleukin-12/23 monoclonal antibody, in patients with psoriasis: 76-week results from a randomised, double-blind, placebo-controlled trial (PHOENIX 1). *Lancet* **371:** 1665–1674.

32. Papp, K.A., R.G. Langley, M. Lebwohl, *et al.* 2008. Efficacy and safety of ustekinumab, a human interleukin-12/23 monoclonal antibody, in patients with psoriasis: 52-week results from a randomised, double-blind, placebo-controlled trial (PHOENIX 2). *Lancet* **371:** 1675–1684.

33. Griffiths, C.E., B.E. Strober, P. Van Der Kerkof, *et al.* 2010. Comparison of ustekinumab and etanercept for moderate to severe psoriasis. *N. Engl. J. Med.* **362:** 118–128.

34. Langley, R.G., S.R. Feldman, C. Han, *et al.* 2010. Ustekinumab significantly improves symptoms of anxiety, depression, and skin-related quality of life in patients with moderate to severe psoriasis: results from a randomized, double-blind, placebo-controlled phase III trial. *J. Am. Acad. Dermatol.* **63:** 457–465.

35. Lebwohl, M., K. Papp, C. Han, *et al.* 2010. Ustekinumab improves health-related quality of life in patients with moderate to severe psoriasis: results from the PHOENIX 1 trial. *Brit. J. Dermatol.* **162:** 137–146.

36. Airoldi, I., E. Di Carlo, C. Cocco, *et al.* 2005. Lack of *Il12rb2* signaling predisposes to spontaneous autoimmunity and malignancy. *Blood* **106:** 3846–3853.

37. Novelli, F. & J.L. Casanova. 2004. The role of IL-12, IL-23 and IFN-gamma in immunity to viruses. *Cytokine Growth Factor Rev.* **15:** 367–377.

38. Murphy, C.A., C.L. Langrish, Y. Chen, *et al.* 2003. Divergent pro- and anti-inflammatory roles for IL-23 and Il-12 in joint autoimmune inflammation. *J. Exp. Med.* **198:** 1951–1957.

39. Ciric, B., M. El-behi, R. Cabrera, *et al.* 2009. IL-23 drives pathogenic IL-17-producing CD8+ T cells. *J. Immunol.* **182:** 5296–5305.

40. Rong, G., Y. Zhou, Y. Xiong, *et al.* 2009. Imbalance between T helper type 17 and T regulatory cells in patients with primary biliary cirrhosis: the serum cytokine profile and peripheral cell population. *Clin. Exp. Immunol.* **156:** 217–225.

41. Berrebi, D., M. Besnard, G. Fromont-Hankard, *et al.* 1998. Interleukin-12 expression is focally enhanced in the gastric mucosa of pediatric patients with Crohn's disease. *Am. J. Pathol.* **152:** 667–672.

42. Cua, D.J., J. Sherlock, Y. Chen, *et al.* 2003. Interleukin-23 rather than interleukin-12 is the critical cytokine for autoimmune inflammation of the brain. *Nature* **421:** 744–748.

43. Shigehara, K., N. Shijubo, M. Ohmichi, *et al.* 2001. IL-12 and Il-18 are increased and stimulate IFN-γ production in sarcoid lungs. *J. Immunol.* **166:** 642–649.

44. Sandborn, W.J., B.G. Feagan, R.N. Fedorak, *et al.* 2008. A randomized trial of ustekinumab, a human interleukin-12/23 monoclonal antibody, in patients with moderate to severe Crohn's disease. *Gastroenterology* **135:** 1130–1141.

45. Gottlieb, A., A. Menter, A. Mendelsohn, *et al.* 2009. Ustekinumab, a human interleukin 12/23 monoclonal antibody, for psoriatic arthritis: randomised, double-blind, placebo-controlled, crossover trial. *Lancet* **373:** 633–640.

46. Segal, B.M., C.S. Constantinescu, A. Raychaudhuri, *et al.* 2008. Repeated subcutaneous injections of IL12/23 p40 neutralising antibody, ustekinumab, in patients with relapsing-remitting multiple sclerosis: a phase II, double-blind, placebo-controlled, randomised, dose-ranging study. *Lancet Neurol.* **7:** 796–804.

47. Dillon, S.B. 2010. New mechanisms and expanded indications for biologic therapies: a perspective on immunology research and development. *Drug Disc. World* **Fall:** 87–93.

48. Nograles, K.E., L.C. Zaba, E. Guttman, *et al.* 2008. Th17 cytokines interleukin (IL)-17 and IL-22 modulate distinct inflammatory and keratinocyte-response pathways. *Br. J. Dermatol.* **159:** 1092–1102.

49. Zaba, L.C., I. Cardinale, P. Gilleaudeau, *et al.* 2007. Amelioration of epidermal hyperplasia by TNF inhibition is associated with reduced Th17 responses. *J. Exp. Med.* **204:** 3183–3194.

50. Katugampola, R.P., V.J. Lewis & A.Y. Finlay. 2007. The dermatology life quality index: assessing the efficacy of biological therapies for psoriasis. *Brit. J. Dermatol.* **156:** 945–950.

Ann. N.Y. Acad. Sci. ISSN 0077-8923

ANNALS OF THE NEW YORK ACADEMY OF SCIENCES
Issue: *Pharmaceutical Science to Improve the Human Condition: Prix Galien 2011*

Development and clinical evaluation of Prevnar 13, a 13-valent pneumococococcal CRM$_{197}$ conjugate vaccine

William C. Gruber, Daniel A. Scott, and Emilio A. Emini

Pfizer Inc., Pearl River, New York

Address for correspondence: William C. Gruber, M.D., Pfizer Vaccine Clinical Research, 190-4202, 401 N. Middletown Road, Pearl River, NY 10965. bill.gruber@pfizer.com

Pneumococcus is the leading cause of bacterial illness in children worldwide. The development, clinical evaluation, and postlicensure impact of the pneumococcal CRM$_{197}$ protein conjugate vaccine, PCV13, (Prevnar 13®) builds upon the excellent safety and substantial effectiveness of PCV7 (Prevnar®) in preventing pneumococcal disease in children. PCV13 adds pneumococcal serotypes 1, 3, 5, 6A, 7F, and 19A to serotypes 4, 6B, 9V, 14, 18C, 19F, 23F in PCV7 to provide comprehensive coverage for over 85% of epidemiologically important pneumococcal serotypes in the United States and throughout the world. PCV13 development required demonstration of immunologic responses to the 13 serotypes contained in the vaccine that were noninferior to the responses elicited by PCV7, and demonstration of a satisfactory safety profile. Studies were also performed to demonstrate compatibility with other childhood vaccines. Now licensed in many countries worldwide, PCV13 shows significant promise for expanded protection against pneumococcal disease in children.

Keywords: pneumococcus; pneumococcal; conjugate; vaccine; infants; children

Introduction

Streptococcus pneumoniae, or pneumococcus, is a bacteria that is major cause of illness in adults and children worldwide.[1] Pneumococcal disease can be classified by clinical presentation (invasive or non-invasive) and by risk factors (age, living circumstances, and underlying medical conditions). The clinical presentations of invasive pneumococcal disease (IPD) include meningitis, bacteremia, and bacteremic pneumonia. IPD is defined by isolation of pneumococcus from a normally sterile site such as cerebrospinal fluid or blood, as well as pleural fluid or peritoneal fluid. Pneumonia without bacteremia is the most common serious manifestation of non-invasive pneumococcal disease and the pneumococcus is the most common bacterial cause of pneumonia in the outpatient setting. In addition, pneumococcal acute middle ear infection (acute otitis media or AOM) is a major cause of morbidity in children.

The pneumococcus is well equipped to cause such human disease. The organism is protected by a polysaccharide capsule, and this capsule has been known to be associated with virulence for over 100 years.[2] Pneumococci can be serotyped by raising antibody to the capsule. Over 90 different serotypes have been identified, but only a minority of these serotypes is commonly associated with disease. Capsular serotype specific antibody in the presence of complement and phagocytic cells can kill the organism and eliminate the disease threat.[3] Prevnar 13 and its predecessor Prevnar have been developed to induce serotype specific antibody to protect infants, children, and adults against pneumococcal disease caused by the epidemiologically important pneumococcal serotypes contained in the vaccine. Prevnar (PCV7) is a 7-valent pneumococcal CRM$_{197}$ protein conjugate vaccine that contains serotypes 4, 6B, 9V, 14, 18C, 19F, and 23F. This vaccine, which was introduced in the year 2000 in the United States and soon thereafter in Europe and worldwide, has demonstrated dramatic effectiveness in reducing the overall burden of pneumococcal disease in immunized children, and has demonstrated the added benefit of an indirect or herd protection effect in

doi: 10.1111/j.1749-6632.2012.06673.x
Ann. N.Y. Acad. Sci. 1263 (2012) 15–26 © 2012 New York Academy of Sciences.

children and adults.[4] In addition to the serotypes in PCV7, Prevnar 13 (PCV13) adds serotypes 1, 3, 5, 6A, 7F, and 19A to provide expanded protection in the United States and globally against epidemiologically important strains. PCV13 has also been developed for adults and has recently been licensed for this purpose. (The reader is referred to the emerging literature on the potential value of pneumococcal conjugate vaccine in adults and a recent review on Prevnar 13 for adults.)[5,6] This review focuses on the clinical development of PCV13 and its promise to extend global protection against pneumococcal disease in children.

Disease burden prior to introduction of pneumococcal polysaccharide CRM$_{197}$ conjugate vaccine

Prior to the introduction of PCV7, the incidence of IPD among children less than 2 years of age was approximately 180–200 cases per 100,000 per year in the United States,[7,8] with an overall estimated case-fatality rate of 1.4% (Ref. 9). The incidence of pneumococcal meningitis in this age group was estimated to be approximately 7–10 cases per 100,000 per year, with an associated mortality rate as high as 8% to 25% (Ref. 10). Among survivors, a significant proportion had serious sequelae including developmental delay, seizure disorders, and deafness.[10] Prior to the licensure of Prevnar, the estimated incidence of bacteremic pneumococcal pneumonia among children <2 years of age was 24 per 100,000 (Ref. 9). *S. pneumoniae* is also a major cause of noninvasive disease in children. AOM is the most common, estimated to occur in up to 90% of all U.S. children by the age of 3 years.[11] with complications including acute mastoiditis, chronic or recurrent otitis media necessitating surgical intervention (tympanostomy tube placement), hearing loss with attendant developmental and language delays. The medical need for a vaccine to prevent pneumococcal disease in children is clear.

Pneumococcal serotype-specific polysaccharide capsule: a suitable vaccine target

Since its discovery, the serotype-specific polysaccharide capsule of the pneumococcus has been shown to be an important virulence factor. It inhibits phagocytosis by interfering with immune recognition of cell wall constituents by complement or antibody and interferes with intracellular killing.[3] Pneumococci that lack a polysaccharide capsule are typically avirulent, because of an inability to resist innate immunity. Work from the 1880s to the 1930s showed that serum—or "humoral"—derived protection against pneumococcus could be seen in the presence of polysaccharide capsule serotype specific antibody, complement, and phagocytic cells.[12–15] Metchnikoff coined the term *opsonization*, from the Greek "to cater a meal,"[12] based on his observations of cellular ingestion or phagocytosis of pneumococci; opsonophagocytosis is now the commonly used term for description of antibody and complement coating of the pneumococcal organism followed by phagocytic cell ingestion and killing.[2] Opsonophagocytic activity can be measured by an *in vitro* assay (OPA) and has been established as a correlate of protection against pneumococcal disease.[16]

Investigators began to develop intervention measures in the early 1900s, first based on administration of serotype-specific antisera raised in horses or rabbits, or a crude whole cell vaccine. Next came a purified free capsular polysaccharide vaccine first used in humans in the 1940s.[17] By the 1970s, in the classic clinical trials of Robert Austrian, purified pneumococcal polysaccharide vaccines were shown to protect against IPD in young adults, and subsequently demonstrated at least some protection against IPD in older adults,[18,19] resulting in licensure of 23-valent purified polysaccharide vaccine in 1983 (PPV). However, the ability of these polysaccharide vaccines to protect young children against pneumococcal disease proved disappointing; the polysaccharide vaccine was not capable of generating a protective antibody response in young children ≤ 2 years of age, who were at greatest risk of disease.[20,21]

The type of immune response generated by PPV conspires against effective protection of infants. Purified PS antigens act as T cell independent antigens and do not recruit classical T cell help, which appears to be particularly important in generating protective immune responses in naive infants and young children.[22–24]

Protein polysaccharide conjugation provides a breakthrough

Fortunately, covalent linkage of polysaccharide antigens to immunogenic proteins was first shown in the 1930s to overcome many of the limitations of polysaccharide alone.[25] Such covalent linkage recruits CD4[+] T cell help, establishes immunologic memory, and induces protective high titer IgG responses with shifts to Ig isotypes of high affinity and functional activity. These linkages were first used to advantage with *Haemophilus influenzae* type b and *Neisseria meningitidis* vaccines. Such vaccines have led to the virtual eradication of *H. influenzae* type b and meningococcal C invasive disease in countries where the vaccines have been broadly applied.[26–28] Therefore, the protein conjugation technology has been used for the development of pneumococcal vaccines. In PCV7 and PCV13, each of the polysaccharides is covalently conjugated to diphtheria cross-reactive material 197 (CRM$_{197}$) protein, which acts as the immunologic carrier. In the 1990s, PCV7 was shown to induce an antibody response in infants and children that would likely be associated with protection in infants and children, culminating in efficacy trials to demonstrate this effect.

Efficacy of conjugated pneumococcal vaccines demonstrated in clinical trials

In a randomized, controlled study of 37,868 children at Northern California Kaiser Permanente (NCKP) conducted between 1995 and 1998, PCV7 given to infants at 2, 4, 6, and 12–15 months of age was shown to significantly reduce invasive pneumococcal disease (IPD) due to vaccine serotypes by 97.4%, and pneumonia by 20.5–30.3% depending on applied diagnostic criteria and population.[29–31] Reduction in acute otitis media (AOM) due to vaccine serotypes obtained from draining ears was 66.7% and tympanostomy tube placement was reduced by 24% (Ref. 32). In a contemporaneous trial in Finland, protection against vaccine serotype AOM was 57% and against all pneumococcal AOM was 34%, based on aspirated middle ear pneumococcal isolates obtained from affected children.[33]

Additional studies were conducted in populations at increased risk of IPD and other manifestations of pneumococcal disease. Protection against vaccine type IPD ranged as high as 86.4% in U.S. Navajo and Apache children less than 24 months of age.[34,35] In children in South Africa, an experimental 9-valent conjugate vaccine, PCV9 (Prevnar serotypes plus serotypes 1 and 5), reduced the incidence of first episodes of IPD due to vaccine serotypes by 83% and first episodes of radiologically confirmed alveolar consolidation by 20% in healthy children and first episodes of vaccine type IPD by 65% in HIV infected children.[36] In children 6 to 51 weeks old in The Gambia, 9vPnC reduced first episodes of radiologic pneumonia by 37%, vaccine serotype IPD by 77%, and strikingly, all-cause mortality by 16% (Ref. 37). The dramatic nature of these effects led to rapid adoption of PCV7 in National Immunization Programs (NIPs) in the developed world, and has lead to advocacy and introduction into developing countries.[38]

Postlicensure observational studies have documented dramatic reductions in national disease burden of pneumococcal IPD, all cause pneumonia, and AOM in vaccinated children.[39–43] Remarkably, in addition to over 98% sustained reduction in IPD due to vaccine serotypes in vaccinated children, PCV7 also has demonstrated indirect protection exceeding 90% in unvaccinated children and adults, including the elderly.[4] This "herd protection" effect is presumed due to elimination of pneumococcal carriage and spread of vaccine serotypes in immunized children, and has been observed to have health and economic benefits that equal or exceed those of vaccinated children.[44]

Despite the impressive impact that PCV7 has had in reducing pneumococcal disease, a significant global burden remains. The reduction in vaccine serotype IPD in young children in the United States is associated with an approximate 75% reduction in overall IPD compared to the period before introduction of this vaccine into the United States immunization schedule. Six additional vaccine serotypes were added to PCV7 to address the majority of the remaining 25% of residual disease in the United States and to expand coverage of pneumococcal infections in different regions of the world. The six additional serotypes include types 1 and 5 (significant causes of sporadic epidemic disease),[45] type 3 (a major cause of pneumococcal disease including necrotizing pneumonia),[46–48] type 6A (a significant cause of AOM and IPD for which serotype 6B in PCV7 provides only partial protection),[4] type 7F (responsible for a significant proportion of residual IPD in United States),[4] and type 19A (the most frequent cause of IPD in the United States, after PCV introduction, and commonly antibiotic resistant).[4,49–53] Taken together, the six newly added serotypes are responsible for approximately 50–65% of the residual IPD cases occurring among children targeted for vaccination in the United States. These additional serotypes should also cover 85% or more of IPD cases in children less than 5 years of age in Europe and much of the developing world, as documented by surveillance studies performed before the introduction of PCV7.[54,55]

Composition of PCV13 and determination of dose

PCV13 is a sterile suspension of pneumococcal capsular polysaccharides of serotypes 1, 3, 4, 5, 6A, 6B, 7F, 9V, 14, 18C, 19A, 19F, and 23F, individually conjugated to the nontoxic variant of diphtheria toxin, CRM$_{197}$ protein, as in PCV7 and adsorbed to aluminum phosphate.

A dosage of 2.2 μg per serotype polysaccharide, except for serotype 6B (dosage 4.4 μg), was selected for PCV7. Based on high efficacy demonstrated in the NCKP study, and effectiveness against all PCV7 serotypes in postlicensure studies, the same dosage was maintained for the Prevnar serotypes in PCV13 and the 2.2 μg dosage was selected for the additional serotypes. Aluminum phosphate assures robustness of manufacturing and acts as an adjuvant, presumably by serving as a depot for antigen and enhancing uptake by antigen presenting cells for presentation of the protein component to CD4$^+$ T helper cells.[56,57]

Defining the path for evaluation of PCV13

Given the availability of the demonstrably effective PCV7, a clinical trial to assess PCV13 efficacy against IPD or AOM using an unvaccinated control group was not judged ethically acceptable. In addition, the large study sizes that would be required to compare culture confirmed efficacy of PCV13 against IPD or AOM to that of PCV7 was not possible. However, since protection against pneumococcal disease after PCV7 is mediated by the opsonophagocytic capacity of type-specific pneumococcal capsular antibodies, the immune response induced by PCV13 compared to PCV7 was considered an appropriate measure to predict protective efficacy of the vaccine. The World Health Organization (WHO) issued a series of technical reports[58] that describe a standardized enzyme-linked immunosorbent assay (ELISA) for measurement of anticapsular polysaccharide IgG concentrations. The reports recommend a single ELISA IgG antibody concentration of 0.35 μg/mL, measured 1 month after the infant vaccination se-

ries, as a reference antibody concentration for assessment of vaccine efficacy against IPD in infants and young children, and as a primary endpoint to evaluate the noninferiority of new pneumococcal conjugate vaccine formulations compared with PCV7.[58] This antibody concentration value was derived from a meta-analysis of efficacy trials that had been performed with PCV7 and PCV9.[29,34,36,59,60] The 0.35 μg IgG antibody concentration in and of itself does not provide direct information on the functional activity of the antibody response, perhaps best evidenced by the failure of type 19F in PCV7 to provide protection against 19A,[4] despite high IgG responses to the latter. Therefore, functional antibody responses as determined by OPA were judged important additional measures to assess the likelihood of protection.[58]

Therefore, by agreement with regulatory agencies, PCV13 was compared with PCV7 in a series of formal noninferiority studies in infants and toddlers to assess the vaccine-elicited immune responses as measured by the proportion of responders with serotype specific antipolysaccharide IgG ELISA values ≥ 0.35 μg/mL. The noninferiority of the responses was also assessed by comparing the IgG geometric mean concentrations (GMCs). The noninferiority analyses were performed for each of the seven serotypes in common to both vaccines. For the six additional serotypes in PCV13, noninferiority was assessed by comparison to the lowest response among the seven PCV7 serotypes in the PCV7 recipients. In addition, OPA responses after PCV7 and PCV13 were compared to assess functional activity of immune response.

The PCV13 clinical development program

The PCV13 Biological License Application submitted for U.S. licensure included 4700 infants who received at least one dose of PCV13 and 354 older infants and young children. After demonstration of satisfactory safety and immune response in early phase trials in adults and children,[61,62] a series of phase 3 clinical studies were performed that, in addition to establishing the immunological noninferiority of PCV13 compared to PCV7, also comprehensively assessed the vaccine's safety profile, established that coadministration of PCV13 does not interfere with the immune responses elicited by other common childhood vaccines, and established that PCV13 could be manufactured using the

Table 1. Immune responses to the seven common serotypes after the infant vaccination series and toddler dose

Immune measurement	Group	4		6B		9V		14		18C		19F		23F	
Infant series															
% Responders by antipolysaccharide IgG (95%CI)[a]	PCV13	94.4	(90.9, 96.9)[b]	87.3	(82.5, 91.1)	90.5	(86.2, 93.8)	97.6	(94.9, 99.1)	96.8	(93.8, 98.6)	98.0	(95.4, 99.4)	90.5	(86.2, 93.8)
	PCV7	98.0	(95.4, 99.4)	92.8	(88.9, 95.7)	98.4	(96.0, 99.6)	97.2	(94.4, 98.9)	98.4	(96.0, 99.6)	97.6	(94.9, 99.1)	94.0	(90.4, 96.6)
Antipolysaccharide IgG GMC (95%CI) ig/mL[c]	PCV13	1.31	(1.19, 1.45)[d]	2.10	(1.77, 2.49)	0.98	(0.89, 1.08)	4.74	(4.18, 5.39)	1.37	(1.24, 1.52)	1.85	(1.69, 2.04)	1.33	(1.17, 1.51)
	PCV7	1.93	(1.75, 2.13)	3.14	(2.64, 3.74)	1.40	(1.27, 1.55)	5.67	(5.02, 6.40)	1.79	(1.63, 1.96)	2.24	(2.01, 2.50)	1.90	(1.68, 2.15)
Toddler dose															
Antipolysaccharide IgG GMC (95%CI) ig/mL[c]	PCV13	3.73	(3.28, 4.24)[d]	11.53	(9.99, 13.30)	2.62	(2.34, 2.94)	9.11	(7.95, 10.45)	3.20	(2.82, 3.64)	6.60	(5.85, 7.44)	5.07	(4.41, 5.83)
	PCV7	5.49	(4.91, 6.13)	15.63	(13.80, 17.69)	3.63	(3.25, 4.05)	12.72	(11.22, 14.41)	4.70	(4.18, 5.28)	5.60	(4.87, 6.43)	7.84	(6.91, 8.90)

[a]Proportion of subjects with antipolysaccharide IgG concentrations ≥ 0.35 μg/mL (see the text).
[b]Exact two-sided confidence interval (CI) based upon the observed proportion of subjects.
[c]GMCs were calculated by using all subjects with available data for the specified blood draw.
[d]CIs are back transformations of a CI based on the Student t distribution for the mean logarithm of the concentrations.
Adapted from Yeh *et al.*[63]

intended commercial scale of production to yield vaccine preparations that consistently elicit the desired immune responses.[63–69]

In the U.S. pivotal noninferiority comparison trial, PCV13 or PCV7 vaccinations were given at 2, 4, 6, and 12–15 months of age.[63] For the seven common serotypes, the noninferiority primary criterion (proportion of antipolysaccharide responders ≥ 0.35 μg/mL) was met for the majority of serotypes, and, for all serotypes using the GMC ratio criterion after the infant series (Table 1). For the six additional serotypes, all postinfant series noninferiority criteria were met, except for serotype 3, when responses were compared to the lowest serotype response (6B) following PCV7 administration. Antibody concentrations to the six additional serotypes, including serotype 3, were significantly higher in PCV13 when compared directly to responses in the PCV7 recipients. (Table 2). Higher antibody levels were achieved

after the toddler dose compared with those after the infant immunization series for all serotypes (Tables 1 and 2).

Serotype-specific capsular polysaccharide binding IgG as measured by ELISA is necessary, but not alone sufficient for protection against individual pneumococcal serotypes. As noted above, antibody must demonstrate functional activity that leads to phagocytosis and killing of the bacterium. For example, the data in Table 1 show that PCV7 elicits substantial levels of antipolysaccharide IgG responses to the added serotypes 5, 6A, and 19A. Yet, surveillance data obtained after the introduction of PCV7 indicates that the vaccine exhibits partial effectiveness against serotype 6A, but no efficacy against serotypes 5 or 19A.[4] Therefore, the functional OPA responses to each of the PCV13 serotypes were determined across the pivotal noninferiority study and additional comparative phase 3 studies, and the

Table 2. Immune responses to the six additional serotypes after the infant vaccination series and toddler dose

Immune measurement	Group	1		3		5		6A		7F		19A	
Infant series													
% Responders by antipolysaccharide IgG (95%CI)[a]	PCV13	95.6	(92.3, 97.8)[b]	63.5	(57.1, 69.4)	89.7	(85.2, 93.1)	96.0	(92.8, 98.1)	98.4	(96.0, 99.6)	98.4	(96.0, 99.6)
	PCV7	1.6	(0.4, 4.1)	4.6	(2.3, 8.0)	31.0	(24.6, 37.9)	42.5	(36.2, 49.0)	2.8	(1.1, 5.7)	86.6	(81.6, 90.6)
Antipolysaccharide IgG GMC (μg/mL)[c]	PCV13	2.03	(1.78, 2.32)[d]	0.49	(0.43, 0.55)	1.33	(1.18, 1.50)	2.19	(1.93, 2.48)	2.57	(2.28, 2.89)	2.07	(1.87, 2.30)
	PCV7	0.02	(0.02, 0.03)	0.04	(0.03, 0.04)	0.20	(0.16, 0.24)	0.25	(0.21, 0.29)	0.04	(0.03, 0.04)	0.89	(0.79, 0.99)
Toddler dose													
Antipolysaccharide IgG GMC (μg/mL)[c]	PCV13	5.06	(4.43, 5.80)[d]	0.94	(0.83, 1.05)	3.72	(3.31, 4.18)	8.20	(7.30, 9.20)	5.67	(5.01, 6.42)	8.55	(7.64, 9.56)
	PCV7	0.03	(0.03, 0.03)	0.07	(0.05, 0.08)	0.55	(0.47, 0.64)	1.87	(1.60, 2.19)	0.05	(0.04, 0.05)	3.54	(3.15, 3.98)

[a]Proportion of subjects with antipolysaccharide IgG concentrations ≥0.35 μg/mL (see the text).
[b]Exact two-sided confidence interval (CI) based upon the observed proportion of subjects.
[c]GMCs were calculated by using all subjects with available data for the specified blood draw.
[d]CIs are back transformations of a CI based on the Student t distribution for the mean logarithm of the concentrations.
Adapted from Yeh *et al.*[63]

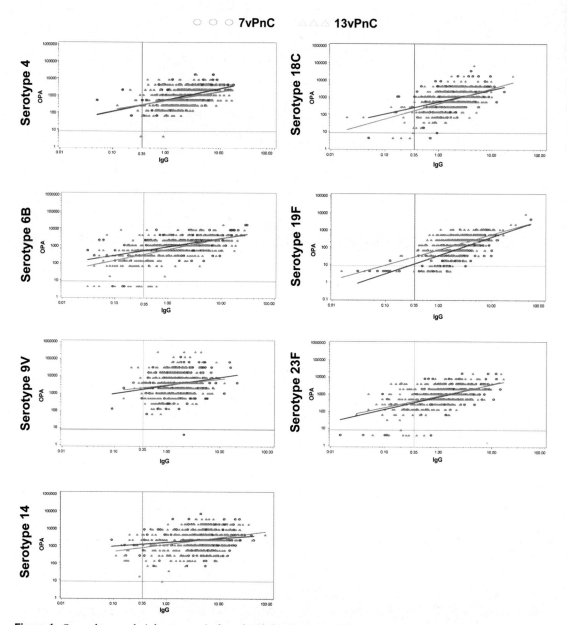

Figure 1. Concordance analysis between antipolysaccharide-binding IgG and functional OPA responses for the seven common serotypes. Shown are postinfant series data from samples with IgG concentrations (*x*-axis) and OPA titers (*y*-axis). PCV13 or PCV7 recipient data are represented. Vertical lines denote IgG reference concentrations; horizontal lines denote OPA responder titer.

association between serotype-specific IgG and OPA responses was assessed.

For each serotype, these associations are presented in Figures 1 and 2. Each panel presents data for a single PCV13 serotype and incorporates data obtained after the infant series in all studies for which both IgG concentrations and OPA titers were determined. Each symbol represents data from a single study subject, either a recipient of PCV7 (red circles) or a recipient of PCV13 (blue triangles). IgG concentration values are plotted on the *x*-axis and OPA titers are on the *y*-axis on the log(e)-scale. The vertical line designates the antipolysaccharide IgG concentrations of 0.35 μg/mL used as the primary comparator point for assessment of immune responses between the two vaccines. The

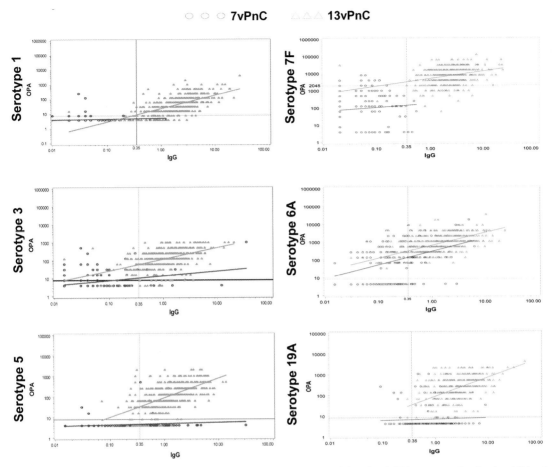

Figure 2. Concordance analysis between antipolysaccharide-binding IgG and functional OPA responses for the six additional serotypes. Shown are postinfant series data from samples with IgG concentrations (*x*-axis) and OPA titers (*y*-axis). PCV13 or PCV7 recipient data are represented. Vertical lines denote IgG reference concentrations; horizontal lines denote OPA responder titer.

horizontal line represents the OPA titer that is the cut-off for a positive OPA response. This value is 1:8 for all serotypes, except serotype 7F for which the experimentally defined cut-off is a titer of 1:2048 (due to type 7F-specific assay characteristics).

PCV13 elicited both polysaccharide binding IgG and functional OPA antibodies to each of the vaccine's 13 serotypes, including the vaccine's six additional types. Serotype 3 exhibited the lowest IgG responses of the six additional serotypes, but the functional antibody response for serotype 3 in the PCV13 group exceeded the response in the PCV7 group by 18-fold after the infant series and 32-fold after the toddler dose; accordingly, PCV13 may provide added protection against serotype 3 disease.[63] In contrast, the antipolysaccharide IgG binding antibodies elicited by PCV7 against the PCV13 addi-

tional types 5, 6A, and 19A are associated with low or negligible OPA responses, consistent with limited or no protection against these serotypes after PCV7. Therefore, PCV13 elicits an immune response that is likely to extend protection to include not only the serotypes covered by PCV7 but also the six additional serotypes in PCV13.

Additional evaluations of the PCV13 immune response

On occasion, administration of pediatric vaccines concomitantly at the same visit has been associated with reduced responses to one or more vaccine antigens. Therefore, the PCV13 phase 3 program contained a series of studies designed to determine the effect of PCV13 on the immune response elicited by concomitantly administered and commonly used pediatric vaccines. No immunological interference was noted,[64–69] providing confidence that administration of PCV13 does not compromise protection afforded by these vaccines.

In addition, it was recognized that it was important to support PCV13 immunization of older previously unimmunized children, as well those who would have received a partial or complete sequence of immunizations with PCV7. Therefore, PCV13 was assessed for immunogenicity in populations of older infants and young children who had not previously been immunized with a pneumococcal vaccine. The immunogenicity data, obtained one month after the last dose for each of the "catch-up" vaccination regimens, showed good antibody responses to all vaccine serotypes, with antipolysaccharide IgG GMCs at least comparable to those achieved after a three-dose infant series.[70] The recommended vaccination schedule for naive older children is shown in Table 3.

Finally, studies were performed to support the transition from PCV7 to PCV13 in infants previously vaccinated with three or fewer doses of PCV7. The antipolysaccharide IgG data from children who received three doses of PCV7 followed by a dose of PCV13 in the second year of life demonstrated that the toddler dose of PCV13 elicited immune responses to the seven common serotypes that are comparable to those seen in subjects boosted with PCV7, and responses to the six additional serotypes that were comparable to the immune responses observed after a three-dose infant series with PCV13 (Ref. 71). These results combined with those of other studies[72] in the program permitted insertion of PCV13 vaccine at any point in the vaccination series, for children previously vaccinated with PCV7, and addition of a single catch up dose for all children who had completed their four-dose series to expand protection to the six additional serotypes.

Safety profile of PCV13

The safety evaluation PCV13 builds upon the favorable safety profile of PCV7 that has been well studied and extensively documented. The safety of PCV7 has been evaluated in several randomized, controlled clinical trials in the EU and the United States, an extension to the pivotal NCKP efficacy trial and a large postlicensure observational study,[73,74] and FDA review of the Vaccine Adverse Event Reporting System (VAERS) database for AE reports associated

Table 3. Vaccination schedule for unvaccinated children ≥ 7 months of age

Age at first dose	Total number of 0.5 mL doses
7–11 months of age	3*
12–23 months of age	2†
≥24 months through 5 years of age (prior to the sixth birthday)	1

*Two doses at least four weeks apart; third dose after the one-year birthday, separated from the second dose by at least two months.
†Two doses at least two months apart.

with PCV7.[75] These evaluations in combination with global surveillance of spontaneously reported adverse events after 195 million doses distributed has confirmed the generally safe and well-tolerated profile of PCV7 for use in the routine childhood immunization schedule.

For PCV13, safety data were obtained from more than 4700 infants who received at least one dose of PCV13 and from 354 older infants and young children. The safety profile of PCV13 relative to PCV7 was confirmed. Solicited and spontaneous local and systemic reactions were comparable between PCV13 and PCV7 groups.[76] Fever rates after each dose demonstrated no clinically important differences.

The PCV13 postlicensure experience

After licensure of PCV13 in the United States, the Centers for Disease Control and Prevention's Advisory Committee on Immunization Practices and the American Academy of Pediatric's Committee on Infectious Diseases issued recommendations for its use in U.S. children. The recommendations state that PCV13 is to be administered as a four-dose series at 2, 4, 6, and 12–15 months of age. Children < 24 months of age who have received ≥ 1 dose of PCV7 should complete the immunization series with PCV13. Children 14–59 months who are fully vaccinated with PCV7 should receive a single dose of PCV13 while children with underlying medical conditions increasing their susceptibility to pneumococcal infection should also receive a single dose of PCV13. Similar recommendations for the transition to and routine use of PCV13 have now been adopted in many countries.

The experience after licensure of PCV13 expands upon the gratifying experience after the introduction of PCV7. To date, PCV13 has been licensed in over 90 countries for use in children, and is now part of over 50 national immunization programs worldwide. Importantly, PCV13 has now become available to 14 GAVI Alliance (formerly Global Alliance for Vaccines and Immunization) sponsored countries, and there are plans to have pneumococcal conjugate vaccine national immunization programs in 58 such developing countries by 2015. In countries with ongoing surveillance such as the United Kingdom, reductions in the seven serotypes in common have been maintained, and reductions in disease to the additional serotypes, particularly type 19A, are beginning to be observed. In early surveillance conducted in England and Wales, type 19A IPD was reduced by 70% (10–90%) after one or more doses, and IPD due to PCV13 serotypes was reduced by half.[77] Given that the PCV13 vaccine is likely to cover more than 80% of disease causing serotypes for most of the world, the potential impact on disease is significant. The previous reductions in pneumonia, IPD, and all cause mortality seen after PCV7, may be expected to be extended as PCV13 comes into common use. After PCV7 introduction, serotype 19A was consistently observed to emerge as the most common pneumococcal serotype responsible for disease across the United States, replacing serotypes eliminated from circulation.[4] The emergence of serotype 19A was particularly prominent in the Alaskan native population, where it was noted to progressively diminish reductions in overall pneumococcal disease to a degree not observed in the general U.S. population.[4,78,79] Serotypes 7F, 3, 6A (including the cross-reactive serotype 6C (see Ref. 80)), less so 1 and 5, emerged as the next most prominent causes of IPD in the United States after introduction of PCV7 (Ref. 4). In comparison to 19A, other uncovered serotypes appear more limited in their ability to fill this new ecologic niche, which may be due to the well-established observation that virulence is an inherent property linked to the serotype specific pneumococcal polysaccharide capsule.[81–83] Therefore, as PCV13 serotypes most responsible for disease are successively eliminated from circulation, remaining organisms may progressively prove less fit as a cause of disease. Ongoing

national pneumococcal surveillance will determine if this proves to be true.[26] In addition, a postlicensure PCV13 safety study conducted in over 40,000 children at NCKP is expected to confirm the satisfactory safety profile of PCV13.[84]

Acknowledgments

This review was sponsored by Pfizer Inc.

Conflicts of interest

All authors are employees of Pfizer Inc.

References

1. WHO. 2004. Global Immunization Data. Available at: http://www.who.int/immunization_monitoring/data/GlobalImmunizationData.pdf. Accessed July 11, 2008.

2. Gray, B.M. & D.M. Musher. 2008. The history of pneumococcal disease. In *Pneumococcal Vaccines. The Impact of Conjugate Vaccine*. G.R. Siber, K.P. Klugman & P.H. Mäkela, Eds.: 3–17. ASM Press. Washington, DC.

3. Kim, J.O., S. Romero-Steiner, U.B. Sorensen, *et al.* 1999. Relationship between cell surface carbohydrates and intrastrain variation on opsonophagocytosis of Streptococcus pneumonia. *Infect. Immun.* **67:** 2327–2333.

4. Pilishvili, T., C. Lexau, M.M. Farley, *et al.* 2010. Sustained reductions in invasive pneumococcal disease in the era of conjugate vaccine. *J. Infect. Dis.* **201:** 32–41.

5. Frenck, R.W. & S. Yeh. 2012. The development of 13-valent pneumococcal conjugate vaccine and its possible use in adults. *Expert Opin. Biol. Ther.* **12:** 63–77.

6. Paradiso, P.A. Pneumococcal conjugate vaccine for adults: a new paradigm. *Clin. Infect. Dis.* (in press).

7. Schuchat, A., K. Robinson, J.D. Wenger, *et al.* 1997. Bacterial meningitis in the United States in 1995. Active Surveillance Team. *N. Engl. J. Med.* **337:** 970–976.

8. Whitney, C.G., M.M. Farley, J. Hadler, *et al.* 2003. Decline in invasive pneumococcal disease after the introduction of protein-polysaccharide conjugate vaccine. *N. Engl. J. Med.* **348:** 1737–1746.

9. Robinson, K.A., W. Baughman, G. Rothrock, *et al.* 2001. Epidemiology of invasive *Streptococcus pneumoniae* infections in the United States, 1995–1998: opportunities for prevention in the conjugate vaccine era. *JAMA* **285:** 1729–1735.

10. Chavez-Bueno, S. & G.H. McCracken, Jr. 2005. Bacterial meningitis in children. *Pediatr. Clin. North Am.* **52:** 795–810, vii.

11. Pelton, S.I. 2003. Otitis media. In *Principles and Practice of Pediatric Infectious Diseases*, 2nd Ed. S.S. Long, L.K. Pickering & C.G. Prober, Eds.: 190–198. Churchill Livingstone. New York.

12. Metchnikoff, E. 1891. Études sur l'immunité, 4e mémoire. L'immunité de cobayes vaccinés contre le vibrio Metchnikowii. *Ann. Inst. Pasteur.* **5:** 465–478.

13. Neufeld, F. 1902. Ueber die agglutination de pneumockokken und über die theorieen der agglutination. *Z. Hyg. Infectkrankh.* **34:** 454–464.

14. Felton, L.D. & G.H. Bailey. 1926. The specific precipitates obtained from antipneumococcus serum and antibody solution by the soluble specific substance of pneumococcus. *J. Infect Dis.* **38:** 145–164.

15. Ward, H.K. & J.F. Enders. 1933. An analysis of the opsonic and tropic action of normal and immune sera based on experiments with the pneumococcus. *J. Exp. Med.* **57:** 527–547.

16. Feavers, I., I. Knezevic, M. Powell & E. Griffiths. 2009. WHO Consultation on Serological Criteria for Evaluation and Licensing of New Pneumococcal Vaccines. Challenges in the evaluation and licensing of new pneumococcal vaccines, 7–8 July 2008, Ottawa, Canada. *Vaccine* 27: 3681–3688.

17. MacLeod, C.M., R.G. Hodges, M. Heidelberger & W.G. Bernhard. 1945. Prevention of pneumococcal pneumonia by immunization with specific capsular polysaccharides. *J. Exp. Med.* **82:** 445–466.

18. Smit, P., D. Oberholzer, S. Hayden-Smith, *et al.* 1977. Protective efficacy of pneumococcal polysaccharide vaccines. *JAMA* **238:** 2613–2616.

19. Austrian, R., R.M. Douglas, G. Schiffman, *et al.* 1976. Prevention of pneumococcal pneumonia by vaccination. *Trans. Assoc. Am .Physicians* **89:** 184–194.

20. Douglas, R., J. Paton, S. Duncan & D. Hansman. 1983. Antibody response to pneumococcool vaccination in children younger than five years of age. *J. Infect. Dis.* **148:** 131–137.

21. Sell, S., P. Wright, W. Vaught, *et al.* 1981. Clinical studies of pneumococal vaccine in infants. 1. Reactogenicity and immunogenicity of two polyvalent polysaccharide vaccines. *Rev. Infect. Dis.* **3:** S97–S107.

22. Harding, C.V., W. Roof, P.M. Allen & E.R. Unanue. 1991. Effects of pH and polysaccharides on peptide binding to class I major histocompatibility complex molecules. *Proc. Natl. Acad. Sci. USA* **88:** 2740–2744.

23. Ishioka, G.Y., A.G. Lamont, D. Thomson, *et al.* 1992. MHC interaction and T cell recognition of carbohydrates and glycopeptides. *J. Immunol.* **148:** 2446–2451.

24. Goldblatt, D., T. Assari & C. Snapper. 2008. The immunobiology of polysaccharide and conjugate vaccines. In *Pneumococcal Vaccines. The Impact of Conjugate Vaccine.* G.R. Siber, K.P. Klugman & P.H. Makela, Eds.: 67–82. ASM Press. Washington, DC.

25. Avery, O.T. Goebel. 1931. Chemo-immunological studies on conjugated carbohydrate-proteins. V. The immunological specificity of an antigen prepared by combining the capsular polysaccharide of type II pneumococcus with foreign protein. *J. Exp. Med.* **54:** 419–426.

26. Active Bacterial Core Surveillance. U.S. Centers for Disease Control and Prevention. http://www.cdc.gov/abcs/reports-findings/surv-reports.html. Accessed March 21, 2012.

27. Haemophilus Influenzae: Epidemiological Data. Health Protection Agency, UK. http://www.cdc.gov/abcs/reports-findings/surv-reports.html Accessed March 21, 2012.

28. Meningococcal Disease: Epidemiological Data. Health Protection Agency, UK. http://www.hpa.org.uk/Topics/InfectiousDiseases/InfectionsAZ/MeningococcalDisease/EpidemiologicalData/ Accessed March 12, 2012.

29. Black, S., H. Shinefield, B. Fireman, *et al.* 2000. Efficacy, safety and immunogenicity of heptavalent pneumococcal conjugate vaccine in children. *Pediatr. Infect. Dis. J.* **19:** 187–195.

30. Black, S.B., H.R. Shinefield, S. Ling, *et al.* 2002. Efficacy of heptavalent pneumococcal conjugate vaccine in children younger than five years of age for prevention of pneumonia. *Pediatr. Infect. Dis. J.* **21:** 810–815.

31. Hansen, J., S. Steven, H. Shinefield, *et al.* 2006. Effectiveness of heptavalent pneumococcal conjugate vaccine in children younger than 5 years of age for prevention of pneumonia. Updated Analysis Using World Health Organization Standardized Interpretation of Chest Radiographs. *Pediatr. Infect. Dis. J.* **25:** 779–781.

32. Fireman, B., S.B. Black, H.R. Shinefield, *et al.* 2003. Impact of the pneumococcal conjugate vaccine on otitis media. *Pediatr. Infect. Dis. J.* **22:** 10–16.

33. Eskola, J., T. Kilpi, J. Jokinen, *et al.* 2001. Efficacy of a pneumococcal conjugate vaccine against acute otitis media. *N. Engl. J. Med.* **344:** 403–409.

34. O'Brien, K., L. Moulton, R. Reid, *et al.* 2003. Efficacy and safety of seven-valent conjugate pneumococcal vaccine in American Indian children: group randomised trial. *Lancet* **362:** 355–361.

35. Watt, J.P., K.L. O'Brien, A.L. Benin, *et al.* 2004. Invasive pneumococcal disease among Navajo adults, 1989–1998. *Clin. Infect. Dis.* **38:** 496–501.

36. Klugman, K.P., S.A. Madhi, R.E. Huebner, *et al.* 2003. A trial of a 9-valent pneumococcal conjugate vaccine in children with and those without HIV infection. *N. Engl. J. Med.* **349:** 1341–1348.

37. Cutts, F.T., S.M. Zaman, G. Enwere, *et al.* 2005. Efficacy of nine-valent pneumococcal conjugate vaccine against pneumonia and invasive pneumococcal disease in The Gambia: randomized, double-blind, placebo-controlled trial. *Lancet* **365:** 1139–1146.

38. Pneumococcal Vaccine Support. GAVI Alliance. http://www.gavialliance.org/support/nvs/pneumococcal/ Accessed March 18, 2012.

39. Grijalva, C.G., J.P. Nuorti, P.G. Arbogast, *et al.* 2007. Decline in pneumonia admissions after routine childhood immunization with pneumococcal conjugate vaccine in the USA: a time-series analysis. *Lancet* **369:** 1179–1186.

40. Nelson, J.C., M. Jackson, O. Yu, *et al.* 2008. Impact of the introduction of pneumococcal conjugate vaccine on rates of community acquired pneumonia in children and adults. *Vaccine* **26:** 4947–4954.

41. Grijalva, C.G., K.A. Poehling, J.P. Nuorti, *et al.* 2006. National impact of universal childhood immunization with pneumococcal conjugate vaccine on outpatient medical care visits in the United States. *Pediatrics* **118:** 865–873.

42. Poehling, K.A., P.G. Szilagyi, C.G. Grijalva, *et al.* 2007. Reduction of frequent otitis media and pressure-equalizing tube insertions in children after introduction of pneumococcal conjugate vaccine. *Pediatrics* **119:** 707–715.

43. Zhou, F., A. Shefer, Y. Kong & J.P. Nuorti. 2008. Trends in acute otitis media-related health care utilization by privately insured young children in the United States, 1997–2004. *Pediatrics* **121:** 253–260.

44. 2005. Direct and indirect effects of routine vaccination of children with 7-Valent pneumococcal conjugate vaccine on incidence of invasive pneumococcal disease—United States, 1998–2003. *Morb. Mortal. Wkly. Rep.* **54:** 893–897.

45. Hausdorff, W.P. 2007. The roles of pneumococcal serotypes 1 and 5 in paediatric invasive disease. *Vaccine* **25:** 2406–2412.

46. Byington, C.L., M.H. Samore, G.J. Stoddard, *et al.* 2005. Temporal trends of invasive disease due to *Streptococcus pneumoniae* among children in the intermountain west: emergence of nonvaccine serogroups. *Clin. Infect. Dis.* **41:** 21–29.

47. Byington, C.L., K. Korgenski, J. Daly, *et al.* 2006. Impact of the pneumococcal conjugate vaccine on pneumococcal parapneumonic empyema. *Pediatr. Infect. Dis. J.* **25:** 250–254.

48. Bender, J.M., K. Ampofo, K. Korgenski, *et al.* 2008. Pneumococcal necrotizing pneumonia in Utah: does serotype matter? *Clin. Infect. Dis.* **46:** 1346–1352.

49. Kyaw, M.H., R. Lynfield, W. Schaffner, *et al.* 2006. Effect of introduction of the pneumococcal conjugate vaccine on drug-resistant *Streptococcus pneumoniae. N. Engl. J. Med.* **354:** 1455–1463.

50. Kaplan, S.L., W. Barson, P. Lin, *et al.* 2010. Serotype 19A is the most common serotype causing invasive pneumococcal infections in children. *Pediatrics* **125:** 429–436.

51. Pelton, S.I., H. Huot, J.A. Finkelstein, *et al.* 2007. Emergence of 19A as virulent and multidrug resistant pneumococcus in Massachusetts following universal immunization of infants with pneumococcal conjugate vaccine. *Pediatr. Infect. Dis. J.* **26:** 468–472.

52. 2007. Emergence of antimicrobial-resistant serotype 19A *Streptococcus pneumoniae* – Massachusetts, 2001–2006. *Morb. Mortal. Wkly. Rep.* **56:** 1077–1080.

53. Messina, A.F., K. Katz-Gaynor, T. Barton, *et al.* 2007. Impact of the pneumococcal conjugate vaccine on serotype distribution and antimicrobial resistance of invasive *Streptococcus pneumoniae* isolates in Dallas, TX, children from 1999 through 2005. *Pediatr. Infect. Dis. J.* **26:** 461–467.

54. Hausdorff, W.P., G. Siber & P.R. Paradiso. 2001. Geographical differences in invasive pneumococcal disease rates and serotype frequency in young children. *Lancet* **357:** 950–952.

55. McIntosh, E.D., B. Fritzell & M.A. Fletcher. 2007. Burden of paediatric invasive pneumococcal disease in Europe, 2005. *Epidemiol. Infect.* **135:** 644–656.

56. Gupta, R.K., B.E. Rost, E. Relyveld & G.R. Siber. 1995. Adjuvant properties of aluminum and calcium compounds. In *Vaccine Design: The Subunit and Adjuvant Approach.* M.F. Powell & M.J. Newman, Eds.: 237–238. Plenum Press. New York.

57. HogenEsch, H. 2002. Mechanism of stimulation of the immune response by aluminum adjuvants. *Vaccine* **20:** S34–S39.

58. World Health Organization. Pneumococcal conjugate vaccines: recommendations for the production and control of pneumococcal conjugate vaccines. WHO Technical Report Series, No. 927, 2005, Annex 2. Available at: http://www.who.int/biologicals/publications/trs/areas/vaccines/pneumo/en/index.html. Accessed 27 October 2008.

59. Jodar, L., J. Butler, G. Carlone, *et al.* 2003. Serological criteria for evaluation and licensure of new pneumococcal conjugate vaccine formulations for use in infants. *Vaccine* **21:** 3265–3272.

60. Siber, G.R., I. Chang, S. Baker, *et al.* 2007. Estimating the protective concentration of anti-pneumococcal capsular polysaccharide antibodies. *Vaccine* **25:** 3816–3826.

61. Scott, D.A., S.F. Komjathy, B.T. Hu, *et al.* 2007. Phase 1 trial of a 13-valent pneumococcal conjugate vaccine in healthy adults. *Vaccine* **25:** 6164–6166.

62. Bryant, K.A., S.L. Block, S.A. Baker, *et al.*, Group PCVIS. 2010. Safety and immunogenicity of a 13-valent pneumococcal conjugate vaccine. *Pediatrics* **125:** 866–875.

63. Yeh, S.H., A. Gurtman, D.C. Hurley, *et al.* 2010. Immunogenicity and safety of 13-valent pneumococcal conjugate vaccine in infants and toddlers. *Pediatrics* **126:** e493–505

64. Kieninger, D.M., K. Kueper, K. Steul, *et al.* 2010. Study G. Safety, tolerability, and immunologic noninferiority of a 13-valent pneumococcal conjugate vaccine compared to a 7-valent pneumococcal conjugate vaccine given with routine pediatric vaccinations in Germany. *Vaccine* **28:** 4192–203.

65. Esposito, S., S. Tansey, A. Thompson, *et al.* 2010. Safety and immunogenicity of a 13-valent pneumococcal conjugate vaccine compared to those of a 7-valent pneumococcal conjugate vaccine given as a three-dose series with routine vaccines in healthy infants and toddlers. *Clin. Vaccine Immunol.* **17:** 1017–1026.

66. Gadzinowski, J., P. Albrecht, B. Hasiec, *et al.* 2011. Phase 3 trial evaluating the immunogenicity, safety, and tolerability of manufacturing scale 13-valent pneumococcal conjugate vaccine. *Vaccine* **29:** 2947–2955.

67. Gimenez-Sanchez, F., D.M. Kieninger, K. Kueper, *et al.* 2011. Immunogenicity of a combination vaccine containing diphtheria toxoid, tetanus toxoid, three-component acellular pertussis, hepatitis B, inactivated polio virus, and Haemophilus influenzae type b when given concomitantly with 13-valent pneumococcal conjugate vaccine. *Vaccine* **29:** 6042–6048.

68. Payton, T., D. Girgenti, R. Frenck, *et al.* Safety and tolerability of 3 lots of 13-valent pneumococcal conjugate vaccine in healthy infants given with routine pediatric vaccination. Presented at the 2nd Vaccine Global Congress, Boston, MA, USA, 7–9 December 2008.

69. Vanderkooi, O.G., D.W. Scheifele, D. Girgenti, *et al.* for the Canadian PCV13 Study Group. 2012. Safety and immunogenicity of a 13-valent pneumococcal conjugate vaccine in healthy infants and toddlers given with routine pediatric vaccinations in Canada. *Pediatr. Inf. Dis. J.* **31:** 72–77.

70. Wysocki, J., E.D. Daniels, D.A. Sarkozy, *et al.* Presented at the 27th Annual Meeting of the European Society for Pediatric Infectious Disease (ESPID), June 9–13, 2009, Brussels, Belgium.

71. Grimprel, E., F. Laudat, S. Patterson, *et al.* 2011. Immunogenicity and seafter of a 13-valent pneumococcal conjugate vaccine (PCV13) when given as a toddler dose to children immunized with PCV7 as infants. *Vaccine* **29:** 9675 9683.

72. Frenck, R., A. Thompson, S.H. Yeh, *et al.* 2011. Imunogenicity and safety of a 13-valent pneumocaoccal conjugate vaccine in children previously immunized with 7-valent

pneumococcal conjugate vaccine. *Pediatr. Inf. Dis. J.* **30:** 1086–1091.

73. Black, S. & H. Shinefield. 2002. Safety and efficacy of the seven-valent pneumococcal conjugate vaccine: evidence from Northern California. *Eur. J. Pediatr.* **161**(Suppl 2): S127–S131.

74. Pneumococcal 13-valent Conjugate Vaccine (Diphtheria CRM197 Protein) 30 Wyeth Pharmaceuticals, Inc (Prevnar 13). Vaccines, Blood, and Biologics. U.S. Food and Drug Administration. http://www.fda.gov/ BiologicsBloodVaccines/Vaccines/ApprovedProducts/ucm 201667.htm Accessed March 29, 2012.

75. Wise, R.P, J. Iskander, R.D. Pratt, *et al.* 2004. Postlicensure safety surveillance for 7-valent pneumococcal conjugate vaccine. *JAMA* **292:** 1702–1710.

76. Sponsor Pre-Meeting Package, Prevnar13, VRBPAC, FDA, November 18, 2009, pp 154–211. http://www.fda.gov/ downloads/AdvisoryCommittees/CommitteesMeetingMaterials/BloodVaccinesandOtherBiologics/VaccinesandRelatedBiologicalProductsAdvisoryCommittee/UCM190736. pdf

77. Miller, E., N.J. Andrews, P.A. Waight, *et al.* 2011. Effectiveness of the new serotypes in the 13-valent pneumococcal conjugate vaccine. *Vaccine* **29:** 9127–9131.

78. Singleton, R.J., T.W. Hennessy, L.R. Bulkow, *et al.* 2007. Invasive pneumococcal disease caused by nonvaccine serotypes among Alaska Native children with high levels of 7-valent

pneumococcal conjugate vaccine coverage. *JAMA* **297:** 1784–1792.

79. Wenger, J.D., T. Zulz, D. Bruden, *et al.* 2010. Invasive pneumococcal disease in Alaskan children: impact of the seven-valent pneumococcal conjugate vaccine and the role of water supply. *Pediatr. Infect. Dis. J.* **29:** 251–256.

80. Cooper, D., X. Yu, M. Sidhu, *et al.* 2011. The 13-valent pneumococcal conjugate vaccine (PCV13) elicits cross-functional opsonophagocytic killing responses in humans to *Streptococcus pneumoniae* serotypes 6C and 7A. *Vaccine* **29:** 7207–7211.

81. Sjostrom, K., C. Spindler, A. Ortqvist, *et al.* 2006. Clonal and capsular types decide whether pneumococci will act as a primary or opportunistic pathogen. *Clin. Infect. Dis.* **42:** 451–459.

82. Alanee, S.R., L. McGee, D. Jackson, *et al.* 2007. Association of serotypes of *Streptococcus pneumoniae* with disease severity and outcome in adults: an international study. *Clin. Infect. Dis.* **45:** 46–51.

83. Weinberger, D.M., Z.B. Harboe, E.A. Sanders, *et al.* 2010. Association of serotype with risk of death due to pneumococcal pneumonia: a meta-analysis. *Clin. Infect. Dis.* **51:** 692–699.

84. Postlicensure Observational Safety Study of 13vPnC Administered to Infants and Toddlers. ClinicalTrials.gov. http://www.clinicaltrials.gov/ct2/results?term=NCT 01128426. Accessed March 21, 2012.

Ann. N.Y. Acad. Sci. ISSN 0077-8923

ANNALS OF THE NEW YORK ACADEMY OF SCIENCES
Issue: *Pharmaceutical Science to Improve the Human Condition: Prix Galien 2011*

The development of denosumab for the treatment of diseases of bone loss and cancer-induced bone destruction

Carsten Goessl,[1] Leonid Katz,[1] William C. Dougall,[2] Paul J. Kostenuik,[1] Holly Brenza Zoog,[1] Ada Braun,[1] Roger Dansey,[1] and Rachel B. Wagman[1]

[1]Amgen Inc., Thousand Oaks, California. [2]Amgen Inc., Seattle, Washington

Address for correspondence: Carsten Goessl, M.D., Clinical Research Medical Director, Amgen Inc., One Amgen Center Drive, MS 38-2-A, Thousand Oaks, CA 91320. cgoessl@amgen.com

Denosumab is a fully human monoclonal antibody against RANK ligand (RANKL), an essential cytokine for the formation, function, and survival of osteoclasts. The role of excessive RANKL as a contributor to conditions characterized by bone loss or bone destruction has been well studied. With its novel mechanism of action, denosumab offers a significant advance in the treatment of postmenopausal osteoporosis; bone loss associated with hormone ablation therapy in women with breast cancer and men with prostate cancer; and the prevention of skeletal-related events in patients with bone metastases from solid tumors by offering clinical benefit to these patients in need.

Keywords: denosumab; RANKL; postmenopausal osteoporosis; bone metastases

Introduction

Denosumab is a fully human monoclonal antibody against RANK ligand (RANKL). The RANKL pathway was identified in the late 1990s to play a central role in the regulation of both physiologic and pathologic bone resorption. RANKL binds to its receptor RANK on osteoclast precursors and mature osteoclasts and stimulates osteoclast differentiation and function, and promotes osteoclast survival.[1–5] The first component identified for this novel pathway regulating bone resorption and remodeling was osteoprotegerin (OPG), which was discovered through a genomics-based approach. OPG transgenic mice were born with high bone mass and marked reductions in osteoclast numbers and activity.[6] The ability of OPG to reduce bone resorption and increase bone mass was due to its ability to bind and inhibit RANKL, a cytokine produced by osteoblasts and other cell types. OPG functions as a soluble decoy receptor by binding to RANKL, thereby preventing RANKL from binding and activating RANK[4] and leading to the arrest of osteoclast formation, attachment to bone, and activation, and to osteoclast apoptosis.

The importance of the RANKL pathway in the regulation of bone resorption was further demonstrated in animal models whereby components of the pathway were either genetically ablated or overexpressed, or in some cases both. Ablation of OPG led to increased bone turnover and cortical porosity and reduced bone volume and density,[7] while OPG overexpression led to increased bone mass.[6] Ablation of either RANK or RANKL led to severe osteopetrosis,[1,8] while injections of soluble RANKL led to increased bone turnover and cortical porosity and reductions in bone volume, density, and strength.[9] Early gene knockout studies in mice revealed that ablation of the RANK or RANKL genes in developing embryos prevented the formation of lymph nodes and the early development of T and B cells.[1,8] In contrast, in studies in adult rodents, administration of exogenous RANKL inhibitors, or continuous RANKL inhibition through OPG overexpression did not reduce lymphocyte counts nor impair the host response to various immune system challenges.[10–12] Overall, the data in adult animals

doi: 10.1111/j.1749-6632.2012.06674.x

suggest that the role of RANKL in the adult immune system may be largely redundant with other pathways.[13]

The role of excessive RANKL as a contributor to conditions characterized by bone loss or bone destruction has been well studied.[14,15] A comprehensive clinical development program for denosumab resulted in a robust data set that supported global regulatory approvals of the RANKL-targeted antibody denosumab in the bone loss and cancer-induced bone destruction settings.

Denosumab for osteoporosis

Osteoporosis is a global health problem that affects an estimated 200 million women worldwide.[16] The condition is characterized by low bone mass and weakening of bone structure leading to compromised bone strength and an increased risk of fracture.[17] The World Health Organization defines osteoporosis as a bone mineral density (BMD) T-score of ≤ -2.5, meaning a BMD value at least 2.5 standard deviations below the mean for young, healthy individuals. In the United States, one in two Caucasian women will experience an osteoporotic fracture in her lifetime.[17] Fractures are associated with significant morbidity and an increased mortality risk that may extend for up to 10 years following hip fracture.[18,19] Despite the availability of effective treatment options, many women with osteoporosis remain at risk for fracture. Observational studies consistently show about 50% of patients discontinue osteoporosis treatments within the first year.[20–22] Complex dosing regimens and concerns about tolerability in the real world setting may contribute to the poor compliance and persistence with treatment regimens and the resultant loss of antifracture efficacy among patients who discontinue therapy.[23–25] Thus, despite the availability of generally tolerated and efficacious therapies, osteoporosis management is not optimal and an unmet need remains for affected patients.

To advance the care of osteoporosis, new therapies must have greater antiresorptive activity, which would lead to significant antifracture efficacy; must be well tolerated; and must be convenient to administer so that the efficacy observed in clinical trials can be realized when the product is used long-term in clinical practice. Advances in the understanding of bone biology permit the development of improved therapeutics for conditions that are driven by an excess of osteoclast activity such as osteoporosis. Denosumab's unique, targeted mechanism of action (modulation of the activity of RANKL, a key mediator of osteoclast bone resorption), which results in substantial reductions in bone resorption, and convenient dosing regimen (once every six months (Q6M) by SC injection) therefore have the potential to improve the effectiveness of osteoporosis treatment.

The effects of denosumab on bone mass and strength were tested in animal models of osteoporosis. In mature, ovariectomized cynomolgus monkeys, denosumab treatment for 16 months reduced bone turnover and increased bone mass at cortical and trabecular sites compared with vehicle-treated OVX controls (OVX-Veh).[26] Mechanical testing showed denosumab improved bone strength parameters including peak load (Fig. 1A and B), stiffness, and energy to failure while maintaining normal bone material properties.[26] Bone histomorphometry demonstrated that denosumab inhibited tissue-level bone remodeling at all sites compared with OVX-Veh animals.[27] Denosumab also reduced trabecular bone surface erosion by up to 86% and cortical porosity by up to 72% (Fig. 1C and D).[27]

Denosumab (60 mg administered Q6M) is approved for the treatment of postmenopausal women with osteoporosis at high/increased risk for fracture.[28,29] Denosumab was first evaluated in humans in a trial of 49 healthy postmenopausal women. A single dose of denosumab reduced bone turnover marker (BTM) levels by 77% within 12 hours, and this effect was maintained for up to six months at the higher doses studied.[30] A larger phase 2 trial in postmenopausal women with low bone mass evaluated multiple doses of denosumab given subcutaneously every three months (Q3M) or Q6M, with the primary outcome measure being the change in lumbar spine BMD at 12 months compared with placebo. The 60 mg Q6M dose was selected as the dose for phase 3 trials because no additional pharmacodynamic activity was demonstrated at doses higher than 60 mg Q6M, and the Q6M interval was selected for convenience and potentially increased patient compliance. Subjects receiving continued denosumab for eight years in the extension of this phase 2 trial had mean BMD gains of 16.5% at the lumbar spine and 6.8% at the total hip.[31]

Fracture risk reduction with denosumab was evaluated in a double-blind, placebo-controlled

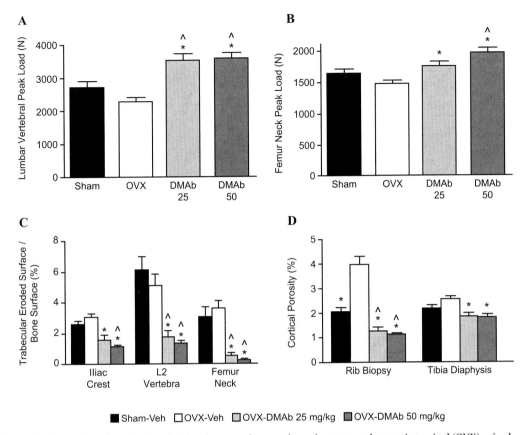

Figure 1. In a study performed using adult female cynomolgus monkeys, sham operated or ovariectomized (OVX) animals were treated by subcutaneous injection with vehicle (Sham and OVX-Veh) or denosumab (Dmab) at 25 or 50 mg/kg every four weeks for 16 months beginning one month after surgery. Compared to OVX-Veh controls, denosumab-treated OVX animals exhibited significantly greater peak load at the (A) lumbar vertebrae and (B) femur neck, (C) significantly lower eroded bone surface, and (D) significantly lower cortical porosity in month six rib biopsies. Data are expressed as mean ± SE, $n = 14$–20 per group. *$P < 0.05$ versus OVX-Veh; ^$P < 0.05$ versus Sham. Figures reprinted from Ominsky *et al.*[26] and Kostenuik *et al.*[27] with permission from Elsevier.

study in 7808 women with postmenopausal osteoporosis.[32] Denosumab treatment for three years significantly reduced the risk of new vertebral fracture by 68% compared with placebo ($P < 0.001$). Denosumab also significantly reduced hip fracture risk by 40% ($P = 0.04$) and nonvertebral fracture risk by 20% ($P = 0.01$) (Fig. 2A).

Reductions in fracture risk were accompanied by significant reductions in BTM levels and significant increases in BMD at the lumbar spine and total hip.[32] Data from this study showed that hip BMD changes at three years explained up to 51% of the new vertebral fracture risk reduction and up to 87% of the nonvertebral fracture risk reduction observed with denosumab treatment.[33] This is a larger proportion

than what has been reported for other osteoporosis agents.[34–36]

Participants who missed no more than one dose of investigational product in the pivotal phase 3 fracture trial and completed the month 36 study visit were eligible to enter a seven-year, single-arm, open-label extension that will continue to evaluate denosumab 60 mg Q6M administration for up to a total of 10 years. Over the first two years of the extension, BMD continued to increase in the long-term treatment group (those subjects who received denosumab in the parent study and the extension, i.e., five years of continuous denosumab treatment) and vertebral and nonvertebral fracture rates remained low (Fig. 2B–D).[37]

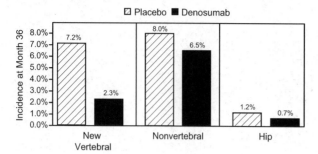

A. Fracture Reduction in Pivotal Fracture Trial

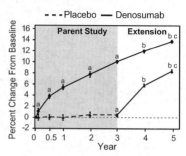

D. Lumbar Spine BMD

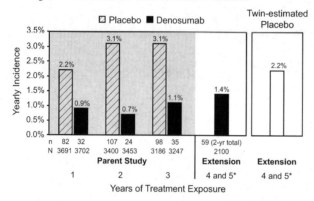

B. Long-term Denosumab: New Vertebral Fractures

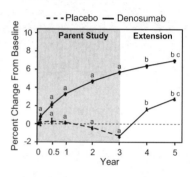

E. Total Hip BMD

C. Long-term Denosumab: Nonvertebral Fractures

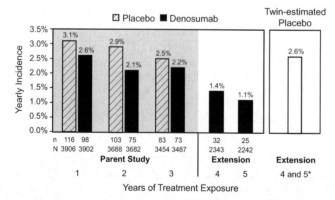

Figure 2. (A) Incidence of new vertebral, nonvertebral, and hip fractures with placebo and denosumab (60 mg Q6M) at 36 months in postmenopausal women with osteoporosis in the phase 3 pivotal fracture trial.[32] (B) New vertebral and (C) nonvertebral fractures by year for placebo and denosumab in the pivotal fracture trial and for the long-term denosumab group in the first two years of on open-label extension. Comparison to a twin-estimated placebo group in the extension phase is shown. *Annualized rate, i.e., (two-year rate)/2. Lateral radiographs (lumbar and thoracic) were not obtained at year four (year 1 of the extension). (D) Percent change from baseline in lumbar spine and (E) total hip BMD over time with placebo and/or denosumab treatment in the pivotal fracture trial and long-term extension. [a]$P < 0.05$ compared with parent study baseline; [b]$P < 0.05$ compared with parent study baseline and extension baseline. [c]$P < 0.05$ compared with year 4. Panels B–E originally published in Papapoulos *et al.*[37] © 2012 American Society for Bone and Mineral Research.

Two additional studies compared the effects of denosumab and the bisphosphonate alendronate on BMD. In postmenopausal women with low bone mass who were naive to bisphosphonate therapy and in those with prior bisphosphonate use, denosumab treatment led to significantly greater gains in BMD compared with alendronate at all measured skeletal sites.[38,39]

Both cortical and trabecular bone contribute to bone strength.[40] Analysis of the distal radius by high-resolution peripheral quantitative computed tomography (HR-pQCT)—an imaging technique that allows measurement of volumetric BMD and distinguishes between cortical and trabecular bone compartments—indicated that denosumab increased cortical, trabecular, and total BMD and improved polar moment of inertia, a surrogate for bone strength, to a greater extent than placebo or alendronate.[41] Denosumab also significantly reduced cortical porosity compared with placebo.[42]

The effects of denosumab are reversible upon discontinuation. In a four-year study in postmenopausal women with low BMD, two years of denosumab or placebo treatment were followed by two years without treatment. Significant increases in BMD and reductions in bone turnover were observed with denosumab during the treatment phase.[43] After denosumab cessation, BTM levels initially increased above study baseline transiently and returned to baseline levels by 24 months.[44] While BMD decreased after discontinuation of denosumab, it remained above the BMD levels in the placebo group at 24 months after discontinuation.[44] In a separate study, histomorphometric evaluation of bone biopsies from subjects who discontinued denosumab treatment for an average of 25 months showed that tissue-level bone remodeling and structural parameters were similar to those observed in a comparator group of postmenopausal women with osteoporosis not receiving treatment.[45]

The pivotal phase 3 fracture trial and its ongoing extension provide the largest body of available clinical trial data on the safety profile of denosumab in the osteoporosis setting. In the three-year double-blind phase, the overall incidence of adverse events and serious adverse events between the denosumab and placebo groups was similar.[32] All subjects received calcium and vitamin D supplements and the incidence of hypocalcemia was low. Certain skin conditions including eczema and serious adverse events of cellulitis occurred more frequently with denosumab than with placebo.[32,46] The overall incidence of serious adverse events of infection was not significantly different between the denosumab and placebo groups (4.1% vs 3.4%; $P = 0.14$).[32] In a smaller phase 3 trial in postmenopausal women with low bone mass, more subjects receiving denosumab than placebo were hospitalized for serious adverse events of infections (4.9% vs. 0.6%, $P = 0.02$);[43] however this has not been observed in other clinical trials with the 60 mg Q6M dose or with the higher 120 mg Q4W advanced cancer dose. In two years of the extension study, exposure-adjusted adverse event rates including serious adverse events of infections were similar to or lower than those observed in the double-blind phase.[37] Since denosumab inhibits bone resorption, certain adverse events that may be associated with reduced bone turnover, such as osteonecrosis of the jaw (ONJ) and atypical fractures of the femur were closely monitored in the denosumab studies. While ONJ was not reported in the pivotal phase 3 fracture trial, four cases of ONJ have been confirmed through adjudication in the study extension.[37] No cases of atypical femoral fractures were reported with denosumab in the double-blind phase of the pivotal trial; two cases of atypical femoral fractures have been reported in the extension study to date.[32,47]

Denosumab for cancer treatment-induced bone loss

Bone loss and fracture risk are also of concern in cancer patients receiving hormone ablation therapy. Adjuvant aromatase inhibitor (AI) therapy and androgen deprivation therapy (ADT) improve recurrence-free survival in patients with hormone-sensitive breast and prostate cancer, respectively, but these treatments increase bone resorption, leading to accelerated bone loss and increased fracture risk. The bone loss that results from hormone-ablation therapy may be the result of reduced estrogen levels. AI therapy reduces estrogen levels directly while evidence suggests ADT therapy reduces conversion of androgens to estrogens. In rodents, orchiectomy was associated with increased RANKL levels in bone marrow,[48,49] and conditional ablation of the androgen receptor increased RANKL mRNA expression by osteoblasts.[50] RANKL inhibition with OPG prevented orchiectomy-associated bone loss in rats.[48] In a recent metaanalysis of six phase 3 trials of postmenopausal women with early stage breast cancer, the odds of fracture increased significantly with longer duration of AI use.[51] Similarly, fracture risk increases by about 70% in men receiving ADT therapy for prostate cancer compared to those not receiving ADT,[52,53] and the effect appears to be dose dependent.[54] As in the setting of postmenopausal osteoporosis, fractures in women with breast cancer and in men with prostate cancer are associated with increased morbidity and mortality.[54–58]

Denosumab (60 mg Q6M) is approved as a treatment to increase bone mass in women at high risk for fracture receiving adjuvant aromatase inhibitor therapy for breast cancer and in men at high risk for fracture receiving androgen deprivation therapy for nonmetastatic prostate cancer.[28] In a study of 252 women with hormone-receptor positive non-metastatic breast cancer (all patients were to be supplemented with calcium and vitamin D), denosumab increased lumbar spine BMD by 4.8% compared with a change of −0.7% in the placebo group after 12 months ($P < 0.0001$). BMD continued to increase over 24 months when significant increases compared with placebo were observed at the lumbar spine and at all measured skeletal sites including the hip and 1/3 radius.[59]

Similarly, in men ($n = 1468$) receiving androgen-deprivation therapy for nonmetastatic prostate cancer, denosumab increased BMD at all measured skeletal sites.[60] In these men, who were all to receive daily calcium and vitamin D supplements, lumbar spine BMD at 24 months, the primary endpoint, increased by 5.6% in the denosumab group compared with a −1.0% decrease in the placebo group. Denosumab reduced the incidence of new vertebral fracture compared with placebo; at 36 months, the relative risk reduction was 62%, consistent with the vertebral fracture reduction observed in the pivotal fracture trial of postmenopausal women with osteoporosis. To date, denosumab is the only agent to achieve a fracture reduction benefit in men receiving ADT for prostate cancer.

Incidences of adverse events and serious adverse events were generally similar between the denosumab and placebo groups in these patients with cancer treatment-induced bone loss.[59,60] Hypocalcemia events were rare and similar between treatment groups. A greater incidence of cataracts was observed in men receiving denosumab compared with placebo;[60] this finding has not been observed

in other studies, including those using greater and more frequent doses of denosumab in a similar patient population.[61]

Denosumab in advanced cancer

In patients with advanced cancer, bone metastases can have significant clinical consequences such as bone pain, pathological fractures, or spinal cord compression that may result in physical and functional impairment, and increased mortality.[62] About 70% of women with advanced breast cancer and over 80% of men with castration-resistant prostate cancer will develop bone metastases.[62–65]

The development of bone metastases is thought to result from complex interactions between cancer cells and the bone microenvironment. Tumor cell deposits that reach the bone secrete growth factors and other factors that result in a local increase in bone turnover. As increased bone resorption occurs, growth factors are released from the bone matrix that feed back to the cancer cells and further stimulate tumor growth. This interplay is referred to as the vicious cycle of bone metastasis.[66] Osteoclast-mediated bone resorption is thought to contribute not only to the bony destruction that occurs in bone metastases, but also the establishment and progression of skeletal tumors. Because RANKL is a key mediator of osteoclast formation, function, and survival,[3,4] inhibition of RANKL decreases osteoclast-driven bone resorption, interrupting the vicious cycle and curbing cancer-induced bone destruction. Furthermore, osteoclast suppression achieved with RANKL inhibition is a rational strategy to delay the establishment of bone metastases.

Experimental data and analysis of bone metastasis samples indicate that diverse signals (e.g., IL-1β, IL-6, IL-8, IL-11, IL-17, MIP1α, TNF-α, PTHrP, PGE2) generated by tumor cells converge on the local bone microenvironment to upregulate RANKL and/or downregulate OPG production.[67] The net increase in RANKL signal to osteoclasts leads to the focal bone destruction typical of bone metastases. RANKL inhibition has been shown to reduce tumor-induced bone destruction and skeletal tumor burden in preclinical models representing numerous tumor types including prostate cancer (Fig. 3).[67–69] In addition, RANKL inhibition has been shown to reduce pain[70] and increase survival[71] in animal models of bone metastases. As would be predicted by an approach targeting the bone microenvironment

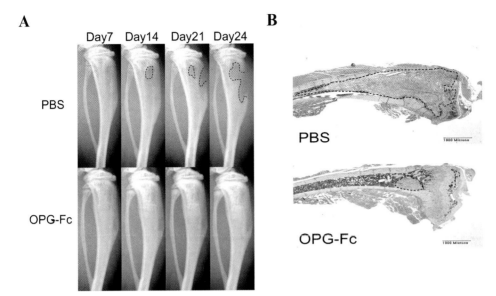

Figure 3. (A) OPG-Fc treatment inhibited progression of PC3 cell-induced osteolytic lesions relative to PBS treated mice. (B) PC3 intratibial tumor burden was decreased in OPG-Fc treated mice. Images from Armstrong *et al.*[68] © 2007 Wiley-Liss, Inc.

and disruption of the vicious cycle, the effects of RANKL inhibition to reduce tumor burden were additive when combined with other pharmacologic agents.[72,73] Through a mechanism distinct from its action in the bone and due rather to the intrinsic expression and function of RANK and RANKL within the mammary epithelium, the RANKL pathway is now known to mediate progestin-dependent mammary epithelial mitogenesis and expansion of mammary stem cells.[74–76] These data suggested the RANKL pathway may also be involved in promoting breast carcinogenesis and metastasis, which is supported by recent data. RANKL inhibition delayed incidence and time to onset of induced and spontaneous breast tumors in mouse models[77,78] and also prevented the metastasis of breast cancer cells to the lungs.[77,79]

Denosumab (120 mg SC Q4W) is approved for the prevention of skeletal-related events (SREs, including pathological fractures, radiation therapy to bone, surgery to bone, and spinal cord compression) in patients with bone metastases from solid tumors.[80] Intravenous bisphosphonates, predominantly zoledronic acid, are effective at reducing SREs. Nevertheless, nearly 40% of patients with advanced solid tumors and bone metastases still experience skeletal complications with zoledronic acid treatment.[81,82] In addition, zoledronic acid has a significant risk of renal toxicity, which can compli-

cate care in cancer patients who are already at risk for renal complications due to underlying disease and critical treatments with nephrotoxic potential (e.g., chemotherapy or antibiotic therapy), and necessitates dose adjustment and continued monitoring of renal function.[83] Further, tolerability of IV zoledronic acid is affected by development of a flu-like syndrome in some patients, particularly after administration of the first dose. Consequently, more effective treatment options with an improved safety profile were needed.

Initially, two dose-ranging studies were conducted to evaluate the ability of denosumab versus zoledronic acid to reduce bone turnover in patients with advanced cancer.[84,85] In one study, patients were naive to bisphosphonate treatment whereas in the other study, patients had received prior treatment but BTM levels remained elevated. In both studies, denosumab reduced levels of the urinary BTM N-telopeptide to a significantly greater extent than zoledronic acid.[84,85]

The ability of denosumab to prevent the skeletal sequelae resulting from bone metastases in patients with advanced cancer was evaluated in three identically designed, randomized, blinded, phase 3 head-to-head studies versus zoledronic acid.[86–88] All patients were recommended to take daily calcium and vitamin D supplements and received standard of care antineoplastic therapies. Denosumab was

Prevention of Skeletal Related Events

A. Breast Cancer

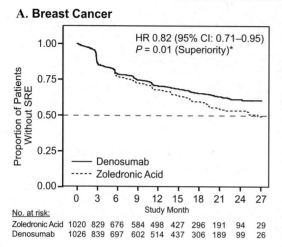

No. at risk:
	0	3	6	9	12	15	18	21	24	27
Zoledronic Acid	1020	829	676	584	498	427	296	191	94	29
Denosumab	1026	839	697	602	514	437	306	189	99	26

C. Solid Tumors and Multiple Myeloma

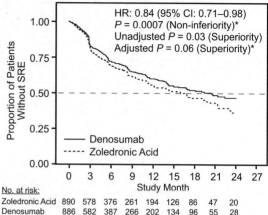

No. at risk:
	0	3	6	9	12	15	18	21	24
Zoledronic Acid	890	578	376	261	194	126	86	47	20
Denosumab	886	582	387	266	202	134	96	55	28

B. Prostate Cancer

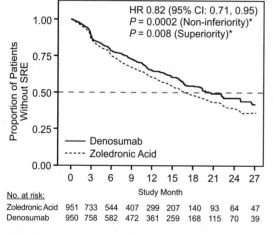

No. at risk:
	0	3	6	9	12	15	18	21	24	27
Zoledronic Acid	951	733	544	407	299	207	140	93	64	47
Denosumab	950	758	582	472	361	259	168	115	70	39

Prolongation of Bone Metastasis-Free Survival
D. Prostate Cancer

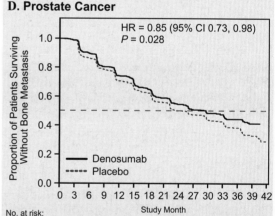

No. at risk:
	0	3	6	9	12	15	18	21	24	27	30	33	36	39	42
Placebo	716	691	569	500	421	375	345	300	259	215	168	137	99	60	36
Denosumab	716	695	605	521	456	400	368	324	279	228	185	153	111	59	35

Figure 4. (A–C) Kaplan–Meier estimates showing time to first skeletal-related event for denosumab (120 mg Q4W) versus zoledronic acid in three identically designed phase 3 studies in patients with advanced cancer and bone metastases with the following populations: A, breast cancer, B, prostate cancer, and C, solid tumors (excluding breast or prostate cancer) or multiple myeloma. (D) Kaplan–Meier estimate showing prolongation of bone metastasis free survival for denosumab (120 mg Q4W) versus placebo in men with castrate-resistant prostate cancer without bone metastasis at baseline. *Adjusted for multiplicity. Panel A is reprinted from Stopeck *et al.*[88] Reprinted with permission. © 2010 American Society of Clinical Oncology. Panel B is reprinted from Fizazi *et al.*[86] © 2011, with permission from Elsevier. Panel C is reprinted from Henry *et al.*[87] Reprinted with permission. © 2011 American Society of Clinical Oncology. Panel D is reprinted from Smith *et al.*[61] © 2012, with permission from Elsevier.

superior to zoledronic acid in reducing the risk of a first (HR = 0.83 [95% CI: 0.76 to 0.90]; $P < 0.0001$) and multiple SREs (RR = 0.82 [95% CI: 0.75 to 0.89]; $P < 0.0001$) in a prespecified combined analysis of data from the three studies.[89] Denosumab was also superior to zoledronic acid in reducing the risk of SREs in the breast cancer (HR = 0.82 [95% CI: 0.71, 0.95]; $P = 0.0101$ for superiority) and prostate cancer (HR = 0.82 [95% CI: 0.71, 0.95]; $P = 0.0085$

for superiority) studies (Fig. 4A and B). In the solid tumor/multiple myeloma study, denosumab was noninferior to zoledronic acid (HR = 0.84 [95% CI: 0.71, 0.98]; $P = 0.0007$ for noninferiority), with a trend toward superiority (Fig. 4C). Among patients with solid tumors in this study, denosumab significantly reduced the risk of first SREs by 19% (HR = 0.81 [95% CI: 0.68, 0.96]; $P < 0.02$).[90] In an ad hoc analysis from this study, denosumab increased overall survival in patients with non-small-cell lung cancer by 21% (HR = 0.79 [95% CI: 0.65, 0.95])[87] while the hazard ratio for overall survival with denosumab was 2.26 (95% CI: 1.13, 4.50) for multiple myeloma and 1.08 (95% CI: 0.90, 1.30) for other solid tumors.

Adverse events were generally similar between the treatment groups in the SRE trials and the safety profile of denosumab was consistent with its mechanism of action as a potent inhibitor of bone resorption. In the three SRE studies, the incidence of events of hypocalcemia was higher for denosumab than for zoledronic acid (9.6% vs. 5.0%);[89] cases were usually mild to moderate in severity and no deaths related to hypocalcemia occurred. In the voluntary reporting postmarketing setting where adherence to labeled recommendations is unknown, symptoms associated with severe hypocalcemia have been reported with denosumab, including rare fatal cases.[80] In the SRE trials, ONJ was defined as a lesion in the oral cavity of exposed alveolar or palatal bone where gingival or alveolar mucosa is normally found, associated with nonhealing after appropriate care for eight weeks in a patient without prior history of radiation to the head, face, or mouth.[91] Events of ONJ that were adjudicated positively occurred infrequently (1.8% denosumab, 1.3% zoledronic acid) and were usually managed with conservative treatment (e.g., mouthwashes, antibiotics, minimal dental/oral procedures) with resolution in up to 40% of cases in the denosumab group and up to 30% of cases in the zoledronic acid group.[91] Median time to resolution (i.e., complete mucosal coverage of exposed bone) was 8.0 months in the denosumab group and 8.7 months in the zoledronic acid group. In both treatment groups, most patients who had adverse events of ONJ had risk factors such as tooth extraction or oral infections, or systemic treatments with antiangiogenics or corticosteroids.[91] As expected, more patients had adverse events related to impaired kidney function and acute phase reactions in the zoledronic acid group than in the denosumab group.[86–88] No renal monitoring or dose adjustment for renal insufficiency is required with denosumab.

Denosumab in nonmetastatic castration resistant prostate cancer

The ability of denosumab to prevent bone metastases has also been investigated in a phase 3 double-blind, placebo-controlled study in men with nonmetastatic castration resistant prostate cancer.[61] Men in this study were at high risk for developing bone metastases based on their PSA level and/or PSA doubling time. Denosumab increased bone metastasis-free survival by 4.2 months compared with placebo (29.5 months versus 25.2 months; HR = 0.85 [95% CI: 0.73, 0.98]; $P = 0.028$) (Fig. 4D) and delayed the median time to a first bone metastasis by 3.7 months (HR = 0.84 [95% CI: 0.71, 0.98]; $P = 0.032$). Fewer patients in the denosumab group than the placebo group had symptomatic bone metastases (10% vs. 13%, $P = 0.03$). Overall survival was similar between the denosumab and placebo groups.[61] ONJ (5% vs. 0%) and hypocalcemia (2% vs. <1%) occurred with greater frequency with denosumab than with placebo, respectively. As in the SRE trials, ONJ could be managed conservatively (e.g., mouthwashes, antibiotics, minimal dental/oral procedures) in most cases, and 39% of cases resolved during the observation period.[61]

Denosumab in giant cell tumor of bone

Denosumab has also shown a benefit in the treatment of giant cell tumor of bone (GCTB), a rare bone tumor with high expression of RANKL. Currently there are no approved therapeutic agents for GCTB making surgery the only treatment option. In an open-label, single-arm study of adult patients with recurrent or unresectable GCTB, denosumab 120 mg administered every four weeks (with loading doses at days 8 and 15 of the first month) produced a tumor response in 30 of 35 evaluable patients by 25 weeks.[92] Additionally, in a second study of GCTB patients receiving denosumab, 72 of 73 (99%) evaluable patients with surgically unsalvageable disease had no disease progression and 15 of 23 patients (65%) with planned surgery at baseline had no surgery over a 12-month period.[93] Denosumab has shown a favorable tolerability profile and is being further studied in patients with GCTB.

Future directions

With its novel mechanism of action, denosumab offers a significant advance in the treatment of postmenopausal osteoporosis; bone loss associated with hormone ablation therapy in women with breast cancer and men with prostate cancer; and the prevention of SREs in patients with bone metastases from solid tumors by offering clinical benefit to these patients in need. The ability of denosumab to treat other patient populations and conditions associated with excessive bone resorption or reliant on RANKL signaling continues to be explored. These include male osteoporosis, bone metastasis- and disease-free survival in adjuvant breast cancer, and hypercalcemia of malignancy (HCM). In a preliminary report, denosumab lowered serum calcium levels to normal levels in 12 of 15 patients with HCM who were refractory to IV bisphosphonates.[94] Additional studies in these disease states are ongoing.

Acknowledgments

This work was supported by Amgen Inc.

Conflict of interest

All authors are employees and shareholders of Amgen Inc.

References

1. Dougall, W.C. *et al.* 1999. RANK is essential for osteoclast and lymph node development. *Genes Dev.* **13:** 2412–2424.
2. Hsu, H. *et al.* 1999. Tumor necrosis factor receptor family member RANK mediates osteoclast differentiation and activation induced by osteoprotegerin ligand. *Proc. Natl. Acad. Sci. USA* **96:** 3540–3545.
3. Lacey, D.L. *et al.* 2000. Osteoprotegerin ligand modulates murine osteoclast survival in vitro and in vivo. *Am. J. Pathol.* **157:** 435–448.
4. Lacey, D.L. *et al.* 1998. Osteoprotegerin ligand is a cytokine that regulates osteoclast differentiation and activation. *Cell* **93:** 165–176.
5. Yasuda, H. *et al.* 1998. Osteoclast differentiation factor is a ligand for osteoprotegerin/osteoclastogenesis-inhibitory factor and is identical to TRANCE/RANKL. *Proc. Natl. Acad. Sci. USA* **95:** 3597–3602.
6. Simonet, W.S. *et al.* 1997. Osteoprotegerin: a novel secreted protein involved in the regulation of bone density. *Cell* **89:** 309–319.
7. Bucay, N. *et al.* 1998. Osteoprotegerin-deficient mice develop early onset osteoporosis and arterial calcification. *Genes Dev.* **12:** 1260–1268.
8. Kong, Y.Y. *et al.* 1999. OPGL is a key regulator of osteoclastogenesis, lymphocyte development and lymph-node organogenesis. *Nature* **397:** 315–323.
9. Lloyd, S.A. *et al.* 2008. Soluble RANKL induces high bone turnover and decreases bone volume, density, and strength in mice. *Calcif. Tissue Int.* **82:** 361–372.
10. Miller, R.E. *et al.* 2007. Receptor activator of NF-kappa B ligand inhibition suppresses bone resorption and hypercalcemia but does not affect host immune responses to influenza infection. *J. Immunol.* **179:** 266–274.
11. Stolina, M. *et al.* 2007. Continuous RANKL inhibition in osteoprotegerin transgenic mice and rats suppresses bone resorption without impairing lymphorganogenesis or functional immune responses. *J. Immunol.* **179:** 7497–7505.
12. Stolina, M. *et al.* 2003. Regulatory effects of osteoprotegerin on cellular and humoral immune responses. *Clin. Immunol.* **109:** 347–354.
13. Ferrari-Lacraz, S. & S. Ferrari. 2011. Do RANKL inhibitors (denosumab) affect inflammation and immunity? *Osteoporos. Int.* **22:** 435–446.
14. Hofbauer, L.C. & M. Schoppet. 2004. Clinical implications of the osteoprotegerin/RANKL/RANK system for bone and vascular diseases. *JAMA.* **292:** 490–495.
15. Kearns, A.E., S. Khosla & P.J. Kostenuik. 2008. Receptor activator of nuclear factor kappaB ligand and osteoprotegerin regulation of bone remodeling in health and disease. *Endocr. Rev.* **29:** 155–192.
16. Kanis, J.A. 2007. WHO Technical Report, Vol. 66. University of Sheffield. UK.
17. Clinician's Guide to Prevention and Treatment of Osteoporosis. 2009. National Osteoporosis Foundation
18. Cummings, S.R. & L.J. Melton. 2002. Epidemiology and outcomes of osteoporotic fractures. *Lancet* **359:** 1761–1767.
19. Haentjens, P. *et al.* 2010. Meta-analysis: excess mortality after hip fracture among older women and men. *Ann. Intern. Med.* **152:** 380–390.
20. Gold, D.T. & S. Silverman. 2006. Review of adherence to medications for the treatment of osteoporosis. *Curr Osteoporos Rep.* **4:** 21–27.
21. Silverman, S. 2006. Adherence to medications for the treatment of osteoporosis. *Rheum. Dis. Clin. North Am.* **32:** 721–731.
22. Siris, E.S. *et al.* 2009. Impact of osteoporosis treatment adherence on fracture rates in North America and Europe. *Am. J. Med.* **122:** S3–S13.
23. Cramer, J.A. *et al.* 2007. A systematic review of persistence and compliance with bisphosphonates for osteoporosis. *Osteoporos. Int.* **18:** 1023–1031.
24. Reginster, J.Y. & N. Burlet. 2006. Osteoporosis: a still increasing prevalence. *Bone* **38:** S4–S9.
25. Solomon, D.H. *et al.* 2005. Compliance with osteoporosis medications. *Arch. Intern. Med.* **165:** 2414–2419.
26. Ominsky, M.S. *et al.* 2011. Denosumab, a fully human RANKL antibody, reduced bone turnover markers and increased trabecular and cortical bone mass, density, and strength in ovariectomized cynomolgus monkeys. *Bone* **49:** 162–173.
27. Kostenuik, P.J. *et al.* 2011. Decreased bone remodeling and porosity are associated with improved bone strength in ovariectomized cynomolgus monkeys treated with denosumab, a fully human RANKL antibody. *Bone* **49:** 151–161.
28. Prolia US prescribing information. 2012. Amgen. http://pi.amgen.com/united_states/prolia/prolia_pi.pdf
29. Prolia EU Prescribing Information. 2012. http://www.ema.europa.eu/docs/en_GB/document_library/EPAR_-_Product_Information/human/001120/WC500093526.pdf
30. Bekker, P.J. *et al.* 2004. A single-dose placebo-controlled study of AMG 162, a fully human monoclonal antibody to RANKL, in postmenopausal women. *J. Bone Miner. Res.* **19:** 1059–1066.
31. McClung, M.R. *et al.* 2011. Effects of denosumab on bone mineral density and biochemical markers of bone turnover over 8 years. *Arthritis Rheum.* **63:** 1107 (abstract).

32. Cummings, S.R. *et al.* 2009. Denosumab for prevention of fractures in postmenopausal women with osteoporosis. *N. Engl. J. Med.* **361:** 756–765.

33. Austin, M. *et al.* 2012. Relationship between bone mineral density changes with denosumab treatment and risk reduction for vertebral and nonvertebral fractures. *J. Bone Miner. Res.* **27:** 687–693.

34. Cummings, S.R. *et al.* 2002. Improvement in spine bone density and reduction in risk of vertebral fractures during treatment with antiresorptive drugs. *Am. J. Med.* **112:** 281–289.

35. Li, Z., M.P. Meredith & M.S. Hoseyni. 2001. A method to assess the proportion of treatment effect explained by a surrogate endpoint. *Stat. Med.* **20:** 3175–3188.

36. Watts, N.B. *et al.* 2005. Relationship between changes in BMD and nonvertebral fracture incidence associated with risedronate: reduction in risk of nonvertebral fracture is not related to change in BMD. *J. Bone Miner. Res.* **20:** 2097–2104.

37. Papapoulos, S. *et al.* 2012. Five years of denosumab exposure in women with postmenopausal osteoporosis: Results from the first two years of the FREEDOM extension. *J. Bone Miner. Res.* **27:** 694–701.

38. Brown, J.P. *et al.* 2009. Comparison of the effect of denosumab and alendronate on BMD and biochemical markers of bone turnover in postmenopausal women with low bone mass: a randomized, blinded, phase 3 trial. *J. Bone Miner. Res.* **24:** 153–161.

39. Kendler, D.L. *et al.* 2010. Effects of denosumab on bone mineral density and bone turnover in postmenopausal women transitioning from alendronate therapy. *J. Bone Miner. Res.* **25:** 72–81.

40. Zebaze, R.M. *et al.* 2010. Intracortical remodelling and porosity in the distal radius and post-mortem femurs of women: a cross-sectional study. *Lancet.* **375:** 1729–1736.

41. Seeman, E. *et al.* 2010. Microarchitectural deterioration of cortical and trabecular bone: differing effects of denosumab and alendronate. *J. Bone Miner. Res.* **25:** 1886–1894.

42. Boyd, S.K. *et al.* 2011. Denosumab decreases cortical porosity in postmenopausal women with low BMD. *Bone.* **48:** S182 (abstract).

43. Bone, H.G. *et al.* 2008. Effects of denosumab on bone mineral density and bone turnover in postmenopausal women. *J. Clin. Endocrinol. Metab.* **93:** 2149–2157.

44. Bone, H.G. *et al.* 2011. Effects of denosumab treatment and discontinuation on bone mineral density and bone turnover markers in postmenopausal women with low bone mass. *J. Clin. Endocrinol. Metab.* **96:** 972–980.

45. Brown, J.P. *et al.* 2011. Bone remodeling in postmenopausal women who discontinued denosumab treatment: off-treatment biopsy study. *J. Bone Miner. Res.* **26:** 2737–2744.

46. Watts, N.B. *et al.* 2012. Infections in postmenopausal women with osteoporosis treated with denosumab or placebo: coincidence or causal association? *Osteoporos. Int.* **23:** 327–337.

47. Bone, H.G. *et al.* 2012. The effect of six years of denosumab treatment on new vertebral and nonvertebral fractures in postmenopausal women with osteoporosis: results from FREEDOM extension trial. Presented at the 94th Annual Meeting of the Endocrine Society, Houston, Texas, June 23–26, 2012.

48. Li, X. *et al.* 2009. Increased RANK ligand in bone marrow of orchiectomized rats and prevention of their bone loss by the RANK ligand inhibitor osteoprotegerin. *Bone* **45:** 669–676.

49. Proell, V. *et al.* 2009. Orchiectomy upregulates free soluble RANKL in bone marrow of aged rats. *Bone* **45:** 677–681.

50. Kawano, H. *et al.* 2003. Suppressive function of androgen receptor in bone resorption. *Proc. Natl. Acad. Sci. USA* **100:** 9416–9421.

51. Amir, E. *et al.* 2011. Toxicity of adjuvant endocrine therapy in postmenopausal breast cancer patients: a systematic review and meta-analysis. *J. Natl. Cancer Inst.* **103:** 1299–1309.

52. Alibhai, S.M. *et al.* 2009. Impact of androgen deprivation therapy on cardiovascular disease and diabetes. *J. Clin. Oncol.* **27:** 3452–3458.

53. Melton, L.J., 3rd *et al.* 2011. Fracture risk in men with prostate cancer: a population-based study. *J. Bone Miner. Res.* **26:** 1808–1815.

54. Shahinian, V.B. *et al.* 2005. Risk of fracture after androgen deprivation for prostate cancer. *N. Engl. J. Med.* **352:** 154–164.

55. Bliuc, D. *et al.* 2009. Mortality risk associated with low-trauma osteoporotic fracture and subsequent fracture in men and women. *JAMA* **301:** 513–521.

56. Body, J.J. 2011. Increased fracture rate in women with breast cancer: a review of the hidden risk. *BMC Cancer.* **11:** 384.

57. Edwards, B.J. *et al.* 2011. Cancer therapy associated bone loss: implications for hip fractures in mid-life women with breast cancer. *Clin. Cancer Res.* **17:** 560–568.

58. Oefelein, M.G. *et al.* 2002. Skeletal fractures negatively correlate with overall survival in men with prostate cancer. *J. Urol.* **168:** 1005–1007.

59. Ellis, G.K. *et al.* 2008. Randomized trial of denosumab in patients receiving adjuvant aromatase inhibitors for non-metastatic breast cancer. *J. Clin. Oncol.* **26:** 4875–4882.

60. Smith, M.R. *et al.* 2009. Denosumab in men receiving androgen-deprivation therapy for prostate cancer. *N. Engl. J. Med.* **361:** 745–755.

61. Smith, M.R. *et al.* 2012. Denosumab and bone-metastasis-free survival in men with castration-resistant prostate cancer: results of a phase 3, randomised, placebo-controlled trial. *Lancet.* **379:** 39–46.

62. Coleman, R.E. 2006. Clinical features of metastatic bone disease and risk of skeletal morbidity. *Clin. Cancer Res.* **12:** 6243s-6249s.

63. Buijs, J.T. & G. van der Pluijm. 2009. Osteotropic cancers: from primary tumor to bone. *Cancer Lett.* **273:** 177–193.

64. Scher, H.I. *et al.* 2005. Prostate cancer clinical trial end points: "RECIST"ing a step backwards. *Clin. Cancer Res.* **11:** 5223–5232.

65. Shah, R.B. *et al.* 2004. Androgen-independent prostate cancer is a heterogeneous group of diseases: lessons from a rapid autopsy program. *Cancer Res.* **64:** 9209–9216.

66. Roodman, G.D. 2004. Mechanisms of bone metastasis. *N. Engl. J. Med.* **350:** 1655–1664.

67. Dougall, W.C. 2012. Molecular pathways: Osteoclast-dependent and osteoclast-independent roles of the RANKL/RANK/OPG pathway in tumorigenesis and metastasis. *Clin. Cancer Res.* **18:** 326–335.

68. Armstrong, A.P. *et al.* 2008. RANKL acts directly on RANK-expressing prostate tumor cells and mediates migration and expression of tumor metastasis genes. *Prostate* **68:** 92–104.

69. Roodman, G.D. & W.C. Dougall. 2008. RANK ligand as a therapeutic target for bone metastases and multiple myeloma. *Cancer Treat. Rev.* **34:** 92–101.

70. Honore, P. *et al.* 2000. Osteoprotegerin blocks bone cancer-induced skeletal destruction, skeletal pain and pain-related neurochemical reorganization of the spinal cord. *Nat. Med.* **6:** 521–528.

71. Canon, J.R. *et al.* 2008. Inhibition of RANKL blocks skeletal tumor progression and improves survival in a mouse model of breast cancer bone metastasis. *Clin. Exp. Metastasis* **25:** 119–129.

72. Canon, J. *et al.* 2010. Inhibition of RANKL increases the anti-tumor effect of the EGFR inhibitor panitumumab in a murine model of bone metastasis. *Bone* **46:** 1613–1619.

73. Holland, P.M. *et al.* 2010. Combined therapy with the RANKL inhibitor RANK-Fc and rhApo2L/TRAIL/ dulanermin reduces bone lesions and skeletal tumor burden in a model of breast cancer skeletal metastasis. *Cancer Biol Ther.* **9:** 539–550.

74. Asselin-Labat, M.L. *et al.* 2010. Control of mammary stem cell function by steroid hormone signalling. *Nature* **465:** 798–802.

75. Beleut, M. *et al.* 2010. Two distinct mechanisms underlie progesterone-induced proliferation in the mammary gland. *Proc Natl Acad Sci USA* **107:** 2989–2994.

76. Joshi, P.A. *et al.* 2010. Progesterone induces adult mammary stem cell expansion. *Nature* **465:** 803–807.

77. Gonzalez-Suarez, E. *et al.* 2010. RANK ligand mediates progestin-induced mammary epithelial proliferation and carcinogenesis. *Nature* **468:** 103–107.

78. Schramek, D. *et al.* 2010. Osteoclast differentiation factor RANKL controls development of progestin-driven mammary cancer. *Nature* **468:** 98–102.

79. Tan, W. *et al.* 2011. Tumour-infiltrating regulatory T cells stimulate mammary cancer metastasis through RANKL-RANK signalling. *Nature* **470:** 548–553.

80. Xgeva US prescribing information. 2012. Amgen Inc. http://pi.amgen.com/united_states/xgeva/xgeva_pi.pdf

81. Rosen, L.S. *et al.* 2003. Zoledronic acid versus placebo in the treatment of skeletal metastases in patients with lung cancer and other solid tumors: a phase III, double-blind, randomized trial–the Zoledronic Acid Lung Cancer and Other Solid Tumors Study Group. *J. Clin. Oncol.* **21:** 3150–3157.

82. Saad, F. *et al.* 2002. A randomized, placebo-controlled trial of zoledronic acid in patients with hormone-refractory metastatic prostate carcinoma. *J. Natl. Cancer Inst.* **94:** 1458–1468.

83. Zometa US prescribing information. 2010. Novartis. http://www.pharma.us.novartis.com/product/pi/pdf/Zometa.pdf

84. Fizazi, K. *et al.* 2009. Denosumab treatment of prostate cancer with bone metastases and increased urine N-telopeptide levels after therapy with intravenous bisphosphonates: results of a randomized phase II trial. *J. Urol.* **182:** 509–515; discussion 515–506.

85. Lipton, A. *et al.* 2007. Randomized active-controlled phase II study of denosumab efficacy and safety in patients with breast cancer-related bone metastases. *J. Clin. Oncol.* **25:** 4431–4437.

86. Fizazi, K. *et al.* 2011. Denosumab versus zoledronic acid for treatment of bone metastases in men with castration-resistant prostate cancer: a randomised, double-blind study. *Lancet* **377:** 813–822.

87. Henry, D.H. *et al.* 2011. Randomized, double-blind study of denosumab versus zoledronic acid in the treatment of bone metastases in patients with advanced cancer (excluding breast and prostate cancer) or multiple myeloma. *J. Clin. Oncol.* **29:** 1125–1132.

88. Stopeck, A.T. *et al.* 2010. Denosumab compared with zoledronic acid for the treatment of bone metastases in patients with advanced breast cancer: a randomized, double-blind study. *J. Clin. Oncol.* **28:** 5132–5139.

89. Lipton, A. *et al.* 2010. Comparison of denosumab versus zoledronic acid (ZA) for the treatment of bone metastases in advanced cancer patients: an integrated analysis of 3 pivotal trials. *Ann. Oncol.* **21:** viii380 Abstract 1249P.

90. Henry, D.H. *et al.* 2010. Delayed skeletal-related events in a randomized phase III study of denosumab versus zoledronic acid in patients with advanced cancer. *J. Clin. Oncol.* **28:** suppl; abstract 9133.

91. Saad, F. *et al.* 2011. Incidence, risk factors, and outcomes of osteonecrosis of the jaw: integrated analysis from three blinded active-controlled phase III trials in cancer patients with bone metastases. *Ann. Oncol.*

92. Thomas, D. *et al.* 2010. Denosumab in patients with giant-cell tumour of bone: an open-label, phase 2 study. *Lancet Oncol.* **11:** 275–280.

93. Blay, J.Y. *et al.* 2011. Denosumab safety and efficacy in giant cell tumor of bone (GCTB): Interim results from a phase 2 study. *J. Clin. Oncol.* **29:** (suppl; abstract 10034).

94. Hu, M.I. *et al.* 2011. Denosumab for treatment of hypercalcemia of malignancy in patients with solid tumors or hematological malignancies refractory to IV bisphosphonates: a single-arm multicenter study. Presented at American Society of Hematology, San Diego, CA, December 11, 2011.

Ann. N.Y. Acad. Sci. ISSN 0077-8923

ANNALS OF THE NEW YORK ACADEMY OF SCIENCES
Issue: *Pharmaceutical Science to Improve the Human Condition: Prix Galien 2011*

Ofatumumab, the first human anti-CD20 monoclonal antibody for the treatment of B cell hematologic malignancies

Ira V. Gupta[1] and Roxanne C. Jewell[2]

[1]GlaxoSmithKline, Collegeville, Pennsylvania. [2]GlaxoSmithKline, Research Triangle Park, North Carolina

Address for correspondence: Ira V. Gupta, M.D., GlaxoSmithKline, 1250 S Collegeville Road, Collegeville, PA 19426. ira.v.gupta@gsk.com

Ofatumumab is the first human anti-CD20 monoclonal antibody to be approved for patients in the United States and the European Union. Ofatumumab received accelerated approval from the U.S. Food and Drug Administration in October 2009 and was granted a conditional marketing authorization by the European Medicines Agency in April 2010 for the treatment of patients with chronic lymphocytic leukemia (CLL) refractory to fludarabine and alemtuzumab, based on interim results of a pivotal phase 2 trial. Preliminary positive results for ofatumumab in combination with chemotherapy in patients with CLL are currently being confirmed in larger randomized trials in both the frontline setting and the relapsed/refractory setting. Ofatumumab has also shown potential in treating B cell non-Hodgkin's lymphoma, such as follicular lymphoma (FL), diffuse large B cell lymphoma (DLBCL), and Waldenström's macroglobulinemia. Additional trials are ongoing to confirm activity of ofatumumab as monotherapy and in combination with chemotherapy in patients with FL or DLBCL.

Keywords: ofatumumab; monoclonal antibody; CD20; CLL; B-NHL

Introduction

Chronic lymphocytic leukemia (CLL) is the most common form of leukemia among adults in the United States, with an estimated 14,570 new cases and 4,380 deaths per year[1,2] and a prevalence of ~105,000 subjects.[3] CLL is a B cell malignancy that arises from the continuing proliferation of B lymphocytes, which progressively accumulate mainly in blood and bone marrow.[1]

In the United States, there are ~454,000 subjects with non-Hodgkin's lymphoma (NHL).[4] Follicular lymphoma (FL) accounts for 22% of NHL cases (~1 of 5) in the United States, representing the second most common type of NHL in this country.[1,5] FL is characterized by cells that grow in a circular pattern in lymph nodes.[5]

Diffuse large B cell lymphoma (DLBCL) is the most common type of NHL in the United States, accounting for 31% of cases (~1 of 3),[1,5] and consists of fairly large cells that are four to five times the diameter of normal B lymphocytes.[5] CLL and FL are indolent B cell malignancies, with slow disease progression, whereas DLBCL is an aggressive malignancy characterized by rapid proliferation.[6]

Waldenström's macroglobulinemia (WM) is an indolent NHL characterized by bone marrow infiltration with lymphoplasmacytic B lymphocytes and production of a monoclonal immunoglobulin M (IgM) paraprotein.[7]

Current options for treatment of patients with CLL, FL, DLBCL, and WM

Current options for the treatment of patients with CLL, FL, DLBCL, and WM include polychemotherapy, immunotherapy, and chemoimmunotherapy.[1] Chemotherapeutic agents include alkylating agents (chlorambucil, cyclophosphamide, bendamustine) and nucleoside analogues (fludarabine, cladribine), often used in combination.[1] Immunotherapy includes monoclonal antibodies (mAb) anti-CD20 (rituximab,[8] ofatumumab,[9] tositumomab,[10] ibritumomab tiuxetan[11]) or anti-CD52

doi: 10.1111/j.1749-6632.2012.06661.x

(alemtuzumab[12]) used as monotherapy. Chemoimmunotherapy consists of regimens combining rituximab and chemotherapy.[8] Examples of chemoimmunotherapy considered standards of care for these patients include rituximab plus fludarabine/cyclophosphamide (R-FC) approved for CLL;[8] rituximab plus cyclophosphamide/vincristine/prednisone (R-CVP) approved for FL;[8] rituximab plus cyclophosphamide/doxorubicin/vincristine/prednisone (R-CHOP) approved for FL and DLBCL;[8] rituximab plus ifosfamide/carboplatin/etoposide (R-ICE) and rituximab plus dexamethasone/cytarabine/cisplatin (R-DHAP) that are recommended by the National Comprehensive Cancer Network (NCCN) guidelines for DLBCL;[1] and rituximab plus either cyclophosphamide, bortezomib, nucleoside analogues, thalidomide, or bendamustine that are recommended by the NCCN guidelines for WM.[7]

A considerable proportion of patients with these B cell malignancies will eventually experience disease progression and/or develop drug resistance. There are limited options for second and subsequent lines of therapy, highlighting the need for new therapeutic options.

Introduction to ofatumumab

Ofatumumab is the first human mAb binding to a novel epitope that encompasses both small and large loops of the CD20 cell surface antigen expressed on B lymphocytes, whereas rituximab binds to the large loop alone (Fig. 1).[13] Ofatumumab can induce lysis of several B cell lines and primary CLL cells, including rituximab-resistant cells.[14] Ofatumumab induces B cell depletion via complement-dependent cytotoxicity (CDC) and antibody-dependent cell-mediated cytotoxicity (ADCC).[9] When compared with rituximab, ofatumumab elicits similar ADCC but delivers stronger CDC *in vitro* and has a greater ability to lyse cells with low CD20 expression, such as CLL cells.[15] Ofatumumab and rituximab were found to have comparable ability to induce lysis of a DLBCL cell line (SU-DHL4) characterized by a high level of expression of CD20, whereas only ofatumumab demonstrated the ability to induce lysis of a Burkitt's lymphoma cell line (Raji), which expresses modest levels of CD20.[14] Ofatumumab is thought to bind closer to the cell membrane compared with rituximab, therefore leading to improved CDC.[16]

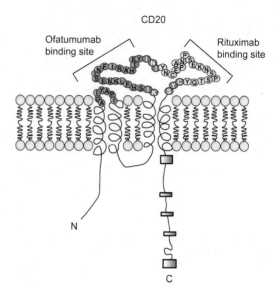

Figure 1. Ofatumumab binds to a novel epitope that includes both small and large loops of the CD20 cell surface antigen, whereas rituximab binds to the large loop alone. Reprinted with permission, Ref. 13. ©2010 American Society of Clinical Oncology. All rights reserved.

Preclinical and clinical data on ofatumumab have previously been reviewed in several publications.[6,13,17–27] A review of the biological properties and clinical activity for the second- and third-generation anti-CD20 mAb, including ofatumumab, has recently been published.[24]

Ofatumumab clinical development in CLL

An overview of ofatumumab clinical development in CLL is summarized in Table 1.

Ofatumumab monotherapy in CLL

Safety and efficacy of ofatumumab monotherapy were initially evaluated in a phase 1/2 dose-escalation trial (Hx-CD20-402) including 33 heavily pretreated patients with relapsed/refractory CLL.[28]

Ofatumumab was well tolerated with almost all (92%) adverse events (AEs) being grade 1/2. Thirty-two patients received all four infusions. The maximum-tolerated dose (MTD) was not reached; the highest dose administered was ofatumumab 500 mg at week 1, followed by three weekly 2,000-mg doses. Fifty-six percent of AEs were infusion-related events, usually reduced in number and severity with subsequent infusions. Fifty-one percent of the

Table 1. Clinical trials of ofatumumab in CLL

GlaxoSmithKline, GenMab, and NCT study numbers	Phase	Therapy	Setting	Status[a]	Efficacy	Safety
N/A Hx-CD20-402 NCT00093314[28]	I/II	Ofatumumab monotherapy	Relapsed/refractory CLL	Completed	ORR[b] = 50% (N = 26) 62% of pts responding within four weeks mPFS = 106 days	MTD not reached (N = 33) 97% of pts received all planned infusions 92% of pts with grade 1/2 AEs 56% of AEs were infusion-related events 51% of pts with infections
OMB111773 Hx-CD20-406 NCT00349349[30]	IIA	Ofatumumab monotherapy	Relapsed/refractory CLL who failed fludarabine and alemtuzumab	Active, not recruiting	ORR[c] = 51% (FA-ref, n = 95); 44% (BF-ref, n = 111) mDOR = 5.7 mo (FA-ref); 6.0 mo (BF-ref) mPFS = 5.5 mo (both groups) mOS = 14.2 mo (FA-ref); 17.4 mo (BF-ref)	50% of pts received all planned infusions Infusion-related reactions: 63% (both groups) Grade 3/4 infections: 24% (both groups)
OMB111827 Hx-CD20-416 NCT00802737[54]	IV	Ofatumumab monotherapy retreatment and maintenance	Patients with CLL who progressed following response or stable disease after ofatumumab treatment in Hx-CD20-406	Active, not recruiting	N/A	N/A
OMB112517 N/A NCT01039376 PROLONG[55]	IIIA	Ofatumumab maintenance versus observation	Patients with relapsed CLL who have responded after second- or third-line therapy	Recruiting	N/A	N/A
OMB114242 N/A NCT01313689[56]	IIIA	Ofatumumab monotherapy versus physician's choice	Patients with bulky fludarabine-refractory CLL who underwent at least 2 prior therapies	Recruiting	N/A	N/A

Continued

Table 1. *Continued*

GlaxoSmithKline, GenMab, and NCT study numbers	Phase	Therapy	Setting	Status[a]	Efficacy	Safety
OMB111774 Hx-CD20-407 NCT00410163 BIFROST[36]	IIA	O-FC	Previously untreated CLL	Active, not recruiting	CR^d = 32% (500-mg group); 50% (1,000-mg group); 41% (both groups) ORR = 77% (500-mg group); 73% (1,000-mg group); 75% (both groups) mPFS and mOS = not reached	All infusion-related reactions were grade 1/2 48% grade 3/4 neutropenia Infections: 38% (all grades), 8% (grade 3/4) 41% nausea (all grades) Thrombocytopenia: 26% (all grades), 15% (grade 3/4) 13% grade 3/4 anemia
OMB115991 N/A NCT01520922[57]	II	Ofatumumab + bendamustine	Untreated or relapsed CLL	Recruiting	N/A	N/A
OMB110911 N/A NCT00748189 COMPLEMENT 1[58]	IIIA	Ofatumumab + chlorambucil versus chlorambucil monotherapy	Untreated CLL	Active, not recruiting	N/A	N/A
OMB110913 N/A NCT00824265 COMPLEMENT 2[59]	IIIA	O-FC versus FC	Relapsed CLL	Active, not recruiting	N/A	N/A

[a]As per www.clinicaltrials.gov.
[b]Assessed up to week 19.
[c]Assessed up to week 24.
[d]Assessed up to three months after last infusion.
AE, adverse event; BF-ref, bulky lymphadenopathy fludarabine-refractory; CLL, chronic lymphoid leukemia; CR, complete response; FA-ref, fludarabine- and alemtuzumab-refractory; mDOR, median duration of response; mo, months; mOS, median overall survival; mPFS, median progression-free survival; MTD, maximum-tolerated dose; N/A, data not yet available; NCT, National Clinical Trial; O-FC, ofatumumab + fludarabine + cyclophosphamide; ORR, overall response rate; pts, patients.

patients experienced infections and 15% had hematologic toxicity.

At the highest dose administered ($N = 26$ evaluable patients), overall response rate (ORR; primary endpoint) was 50%. Time to response was rapid, with 62% of patients at the highest dose responding within four weeks; most of the responses (9/13) were sustained at week 19.

These promising preliminary results were confirmed in a pivotal phase 2 trial (Hx-CD20-406) of ofatumumab monotherapy in patients with fludarabine- and alemtuzumab-refractory (FA-ref) CLL and in those with bulky lymphadenopathy refractory to fludarabine not suitable for treatment with alemtuzumab (BF-ref).[29–32] Patients received eight weekly ofatumumab doses followed by four monthly doses (300-mg initial dose, 2,000-mg subsequent doses). The final analysis, conducted on 206 patients (95 FA-ref, 111 BF-ref), demonstrated the clinical benefit provided by ofatumumab in these heavily pretreated patients with poor prognosis.[29] Eighty-nine percent of the patients received ≥8 infusions and 50% received all 12 infusions. ORR (primary endpoint) was 51% in the FA-ref group and 44% in the BF-ref group. Responses were observed among patients previously treated with rituximab-containing regimens (ORR: 45% FA-ref group, 41% BF-ref group) and in patients refractory to R-FC (ORR: 44% FA-ref group, 26% BF-ref group). Responses were durable, with a median duration of response (DOR) of 5.7 months in the FA-ref group and 6.0 months in the BF-ref group. Median progression-free survival (PFS) and overall survival (OS) were 5.5 and 14.2 months in the FA-ref group and 5.5 and 17.4 months in the BF-ref group, respectively. A *post hoc* analysis of the final data dissecting ofatumumab outcomes based on prior exposure and refractoriness to rituximab revealed that ofatumumab is active in patients with CLL refractory to fludarabine regardless of prior rituximab, as high ORRs were observed in rituximab-treated (43%), rituximab-refractory (44%), and rituximab-naive (53%) patients.[33]

The most common AEs were infusion-related reactions, observed in 63% of patients; nearly all were grade 1/2 and occurred during initial infusions, decreasing with subsequent infusions.[29] Other common AEs were cough (23%), pyrexia (21%), anemia (18%), diarrhea (17%), neutropenia (17%), fatigue (16%), dyspnea (15%), and pneumonia (15%). The most common grade 3/4 AEs were infections (24%), neutropenia (13%), pneumonia (10%), and anemia (5%). On the basis of the positive data from this pivotal trial, the U.S. Food and Drug Administration (FDA) approved the use of ofatumumab in patients with CLL refractory to fludarabine and alemtuzumab in 2009,[9,34] and the European Medicines Agency (EMA) granted conditional approval for the same indication in 2010.[35]

Ofatumumab combination therapy in CLL
On the basis of positive results from single-agent trials and its potential use in combination therapy, ofatumumab was evaluated in combination with chemotherapy. A randomized phase 2 trial (BIFROST) investigated ofatumumab plus fludara-bine/cyclophosphamide (O-FC) in previously untreated patients with CLL.[36] A total of 61 patients received standard FC plus ofatumumab 300 mg (first monthly dose) followed by either 500 mg (arm A, $n = 31$) or 1,000 mg (arm B, $n = 30$) of once-monthly ofatumumab for the remaining five cycles. Complete response (CR) rates (primary endpoint) were 32% (group A) and 50% (group B), with similar ORRs between arms (77% group A, 73% group B). Across all patients, CR and ORR were 41% and 75%, respectively. Although the ORR achieved with O-FC[36] was lower than that reported with R-FC,[37–39] it should be noted that patients included in the ofatumumab BIFROST[36] trial had higher risk profiles (by β_2-microglobulin and 17p deletion) than those included in the rituximab trials.[37–39]

The O-FC regimen was well tolerated, with the most common AEs being infusion-related reactions, all grade 1/2, and mainly occurring during the first two infusions. Other common AEs were neutropenia (48%), infections (38%), nausea (41%), thrombocytopenia (26%), rash (25%), vomiting (23%), fever (21%), headache (18%), and fatigue (18%).

This trial demonstrated activity and feasibility of O-FC for the frontline treatment of patients with CLL, despite the poor prognosis associated with these high-risk patients (64% had β_2-microglobulin levels >3.5 mg/L; 13% had 17p deletion). On the basis of these data, ofatumumab may offer a new treatment option for these patients.

Ofatumumab clinical development in B-NHL

An overview of ofatumumab clinical development in B-NHL is summarized in Table 2.

Ofatumumab monotherapy in FL
Efficacy and safety of ofatumumab monotherapy were initially evaluated in a phase 1/2 dose-escalation trial (Hx-CD20-001) including 40 patients with relapsed/refractory grade 1 or 2 CD20+ FL.[40] Patients were enrolled in four dose levels ($n = 10$ per dose level) of weekly ofatumumab infusions ranging from 300 to 1,000 mg. Thirty-nine patients received all four planned infusions. Treatment was well tolerated; no MTD was identified. A total of 274 AEs were reported in 40 patients; 261 (95%) were grade 1/2. Ofatumumab was considered to be related to 190 AEs (70%), of which 182

Table 2. Clinical trials of ofatumumab in B-NHL

GlaxoSmithKline, GenMab, and NCT study numbers	Phase	Therapy	Setting	Status[a]	Efficacy	Safety
N/A Hx-CD20-001 NCT00092274[40]	I/II	Ofatumumab monotherapy	Relapsed/ refractory FL grade I-II	Completed	ORR[b] = 63% (300-mg group, $n = 8$); 33% (500-mg group, $n = 9$); 20% (700-mg group, $n = 10$); 50% (1,000-mg group, $n = 10$); 41% (all groups, $n = 37$) mDOR = 29.9 mo mTTP = 8.8 mo (all pts); 32.6 mo (responders)	MTD not reached ($N = 40$) 98% of pts received all planned infusions 95% of AEs were grade 1/2 70% of AEs were related to ofatumumab 95% of pts with infusion-related AEs 33% of pts with infections
OMB111772 Hx-CD20-405 NCT00394836[41]	IIA	Ofatumumab monotherapy	Rituximab- refractory FL	Active, not recruiting	ORR[c] = 10% (1,000-mg group, $n = 86$); 13% (500-mg group, $n = 30$); 11% (all groups, $n = 116$); 22% (in rituximab- refractory pts) mDOR = 6.0 mo (all pts) mPFS = 5.8 mo (all pts)	87% of pts in 500-mg group received all planned infusions, 91% in the 1,000-mg group 51% of pts with infusion-related AEs (first infusion), nearly all grade 1/2 36% of pts with infections
OMB113676 N/A NCT01200589 HOMER[60]	IIIA	Ofatumumab monotherapy versus rituximab monotherapy	Relapsed FL after rituximab therapy	Recruiting	N/A	N/A
OMB111775 Hx-CD20-409 NCT00494780 MUNIN[42]	IIA	O-CHOP	Untreated FL	Active, not recruiting	ORR[d] = 90% (500-mg group, $n = 29$); 100% (1,000-mg group, $n = 30$) CR/CRu = 76% (in high-risk FLIPI pts) mPFS/mOS = not reached	96% of pts received all planned infusions 59% of pts with infections (9% related to ofatumumab and all grade 1/2) 28% of pts with infusion-related AEs (nearly all grade 1/2) 29% grade 3/4 leukopenia 22% grade 3/4 neutropenia

Continued

Table 2. *Continued*

GlaxoSmithKline, GenMab, and NCT study numbers	Phase	Therapy	Setting	Status[a]	Efficacy	Safety
OMB110918 N/A NCT01077518 COMPLEMENT A+B[61]	IIIA	Ofatumumab + bendamustine versus bendamustine alone	Indolent B-cell NHL unresponsive to rituximab	Recruiting	N/A	N/A
OMB111776 Hx-CD20-415 NCT00622388[43]	II	Ofatumumab monotherapy	Relapsed/ progressive DLBCL	Active, not recruiting	ORR[c] = 11% (N = 57); 22% (in pts with a response >6 mo from last therapy) mDOR = 6.9 mo mPFS = 2.5 mo	58% of pts received all planned infusions 59% of pts with infusion-related AEs (mostly grade 1/2, 44% related to ofatumumab) 37% of pts with infections (12% related to ofatumumab) 10% grade 3/4 neutropenia
OMB110927 N/A NCT00823719[44]	IIA	O-ICE or O-DHAP followed by ASCT	Relapsed/ refractory DLBCL	Completed	ORR[c] = 61% (all pts); 55% (O-ICE, n = 35); 69% (O-DHAP, n = 26); 59% (high-risk pts with sAAIPI of 2/3, n = 29) mPFS = 9.6 mo (all pts) mOS = 16.3 mo (all pts)	62% of pts with infusion-related AEs, 13% grade 3/4 (first infusion) Thrombocytopenia: 64% (all grades), 59% (grade 3/4) Anemia: 49% (all grades), 36% (grade 3/4) Infections: 25% (all grades), 10% (grade 3/4)
OMB110928 N/A NCT01014208 ORCHARRD[62]	IIIA	O-DHAP or O-DVD versus R-DHAP or R-DVD followed by ASCT	Relapsed/ refractory DLBCL	Recruiting	N/A	N/A

Continued

(96%) were grade 1/2. The most frequent AEs were pyrexia, chills, fatigue, dyspnea, pharyngolaryngeal pain, cough, pruritus, rash, urticaria, headache, hypotension, and nausea. Thirty-eight patients (95%)

experienced infusion-related AEs and 13 (33%) had infections.

ORRs at week 19 (primary endpoint) were not dose-dependent: 63% in the 300-mg cohort (n = 8),

Table 2. *Continued*

GlaxoSmithKline, GenMab, and NCT study numbers	Phase	Therapy	Setting	Status[a]	Efficacy	Safety
OMB110921 N/A NCT00811733[46]	IIA	Ofatumumab monotherapy	WM	Active, not recruiting	ORR = 59% (all pts); 47% (1,000-mg group, $n = 15$); 68% (2,000-mg group, $n = 22$); 50% (pts with baseline IgM $\geq$4 g/dL, $n = 12$)	81% of pts with manageable infusion-related AEs (11% grade 3/4) 41% of pts with infections (mostly grade 1/2) 5% of pts with IgM flare

[a]As per www.clinicaltrials.gov.
[b]Assessed up to week 19.
[c]Assessed over a six-month period from start of treatment.
[d]Assessed up to three months after last infusion.
[e]Assessed after cycle 2 (CT) and 3 (CT + PET).
AE, adverse event; ASCT, autologous stem cell transplantation; B-NHL, B-cell non-Hodgkin's lymphoma; CR, complete response; CRu, unconfirmed complete response; CT, computerized tomography; DLBCL, diffuse large B-cell lymphoma; FL, follicular lymphoma; FLIPI, Follicular Lymphoma International Prognostic Index; IgM, immunoglobulin M; mDOR, median duration of response; mo, months; mOS, median overall survival; mPFS, median progression-free survival; MTD, maximum-tolerated dose; mTTP, median time to progression; N/A, data not yet available; NCT, National Clinical Trial; NHL, non-Hodgkin's lymphoma; O-CHOP, ofatumumab + cyclophosphamide/doxorubicin/vincristine/prednisone; O-DHAP, ofatumumab + dexamethasone/cytarabine/cisplatin; O-DVD, ofatumumab + dexamethasone/vincristine/liposomal doxorubicin; O-ICE, ofatumumab + ifosfamide/carboplatin/etoposide; ORR, overall response rate; PET, positron emission tomography; pts, patients; R-DHAP, rituximab + dexamethasone/cytarabine/cisplatin; R-DVD, rituximab + dexamethasone/vincristine/liposomal doxorubicin; sAAIPI, second-line age-adjusted International Prognostic Index; WM, Waldenström's macroglobulinemia.

33% in the 500-mg cohort ($n = 9$), 20% in the 700-mg cohort ($n = 10$), 50% in the 1,000-mg cohort ($n = 10$), and 41% across all doses ($N = 37$). ORR at week 26 was 60% in the 1,000-mg cohort. Among 14 patients pretreated with rituximab, ORR was 64% across all doses. At a median follow-up of 9.2 months, median DOR was 29.9 months, and median time to progression was 8.8 months (all patients) and 32.6 months (responders).

On the basis of these promising results, ofatumumab monotherapy was tested in a phase 2 trial (Hx-CD20-405) including 116 heavily pretreated patients with grade 1 or 2 CD20$^+$ FL refractory to rituximab monotherapy or rituximab-based regimens.[41] Patients received ofatumumab 300 mg (first weekly dose) followed by either 500 mg ($n = 30$) or 1,000 mg ($n = 86$) once-weekly doses for seven subsequent weeks.

ORRs (primary endpoint) were modest in this poor-prognosis population and did not differ between groups (500-mg group: 13%; 1,000-mg group: 10%; and all patients: 11%). Although response rates (RRs) were low in patients refractory to rituximab maintenance therapy after chemotherapy or R-chemotherapy (9%) and in those refractory to R-chemotherapy (7%), a higher RR was achieved in patients refractory to single-agent rituximab (22%). This suggests that ofatumumab may provide greater benefit in patients with FL refractory to rituximab monotherapy and not refractory to chemotherapy. Median DOR was 6.0 months in both groups. Median PFS was 5.8 months across all patients.

Ofatumumab was well tolerated in this heavily pretreated, rituximab-refractory population. Eighty-seven percent (500-mg group) and 91% (1,000-mg group) of patients completed all eight infusions. Infusion-related reactions occurred in 51% of patients at first infusion, dropping to 8 to 15% during subsequent infusions. Nearly all infusion-related reactions were grade 1/2; only three patients had grade 3 reactions. The most common AEs were infections (36%), rash (16%), urticaria (14%), fatigue (14%), pruritus (13%), nausea (12%), cough (12%), neutropenia (12%), and pyrexia (11%).

Ofatumumab combination therapy in FL

The randomized phase 2 trial MUNIN investigated ofatumumab plus CHOP (O-CHOP) as frontline treatment for patients with FL.[42] Fifty-nine patients were randomized to ofatumumab 500 mg ($n = 29$) plus CHOP or 1,000 mg ($n = 30$) plus CHOP (first ofatumumab dose of 300 mg in both arms).

ORRs (primary endpoint) were high and similar between groups: 90% (500-mg group) and 100% (1,000-mg group). Ofatumumab maintained high activity across all Follicular Lymphoma International Prognostic Index (FLIPI) risk groups, especially in patients with high-risk FLIPI scores with CR/unconfirmed CR rates of 76%.

The O-CHOP regimen was well tolerated. Ninety-six percent of patients completed all six cycles. The most common all-grade AEs were infections (59%), alopecia (48%), fatigue (38%), nausea (38%), urticaria (33%), leukopenia (31%), constipation (29%), rash (29%), diarrhea (28%), infusion-related reactions (28%), neutropenia (28%), dyspnea (26%), polyneuropathy (26%), pharyngolaryngeal pain (22%), and pyrexia (22%). Infections considered ofatumumab-related were reported in only 9% of patients and all were grade 1/2. Infusion-related reactions were nearly all grade 1/2 and decreased in incidence with continued therapy.

Ofatumumab monotherapy in DLBCL

Efficacy and safety of ofatumumab monotherapy were initially evaluated in a phase 2 trial (Hx-CD20-415) including 81 heavily pretreated patients with CD20$^+$ relapsed/progressive DLBCL after failing autologous stem cell transplantation (ASCT) or ineligible for ASCT.[43] Patients received ofatumumab 300 mg (first weekly dose) followed by 1,000 mg once-weekly doses for seven subsequent weeks.

The ORR (primary endpoint) was 11% in 57 evaluable patients. Incomplete data collection prohibited primary endpoint assessment in 24 patients. RR in patients who had a response lasting >6 months to their last therapy was high (22%), suggesting that responses to ofatumumab may be influenced by patients' response to their latest treatment. Among 25 patients with prior ASCT, RR was 8%; among 56 patients who did not undergo ASCT,

RR was 13%. Median DOR was 6.9 months and median PFS was 2.5 months.

Ofatumumab was well tolerated in these heavily pretreated patients; 58% of patients completed all eight planned infusions. The most common all-grade AEs were infusion-related events (59%), infections (37%), diarrhea (17%), fatigue (15%), peripheral edema (15%), neutropenia (14%), abdominal pain (12%), constipation (12%), nausea (12%), pyrexia (11%), anemia (11%), leukopenia (11%), dyspnea (10%), and anorexia (10%). Infusion-related reactions, predominantly grade 1/2, occurred primarily at first infusion (40% of patients) and decreased during subsequent infusions. Infusion-related reactions considered ofatumumab-related were reported in 44% of patients at any infusion. Infections were mostly mild, with grade ≥3 infections observed in 6% of patients; infections considered ofatumumab-related were reported in 12% of patients.

Ofatumumab combination therapy in DLBCL

Ofatumumab was evaluated in combination with chemotherapy in DLBCL. A phase 2 trial (OMB110927) investigated ofatumumab plus salvage ICE or DHAP (O-ICE, O-DHAP) in 61 patients with relapsed/refractory aggressive B cell lymphoma before ASCT, including DLBCL ($n = 47$), transformed low-grade FL ($n = 12$), and grade 3b FL ($n = 2$).[44] All patients had previously received first-line therapy of rituximab plus anthracycline-based chemotherapy. Thirty-five patients received O-ICE and 26 received O-DHAP. Ofatumumab was initially administered as 300 mg on day 1 and 1,000 mg on day 8 of the first 21-day cycle, then 1,000 mg only on day 1 of the remaining two cycles; the initial 300-mg dose was changed to 1,000 mg by protocol amendment after 21 patients had been treated.

ORR (primary endpoint) was 61% across 59 evaluable patients (55% O-ICE group, 69% O-DHAP group). ORR was particularly promising (59%) in high-risk patients with second-line age-adjusted International Prognostic Index (sAAIPI) of 2/3 ($n = 29$). Median PFS and OS were 9.6 months and 16.3 months, respectively. ORR achieved with O-DHAP compared favorably with ORR reported with R-DHAP in patients who had failed rituximab plus anthracycline-based chemotherapy in the CORAL trial.[45]

Ofatumumab was well tolerated, with no unexpected toxicity. Eighty percent of patients in the O-ICE group and 92% in the O-DHAP group received all planned infusions. Stem cell mobilization was performed in 45 patients and in only two cases was the number of cells collected below the amount required for ASCT. The most common all-grade AEs were infusion-related reactions (62% at first infusion, 49% in subsequent infusions), thrombocytopenia (64%), anemia (49%), infections (25%), increased creatinine (23%), and febrile neutropenia (15%).

Ofatumumab monotherapy in WM

Efficacy and safety of ofatumumab monotherapy were evaluated in a phase 2 trial (OMB110921) that treated 37 patients with WM with a first weekly dose of ofatumumab 300 mg followed by either three weekly 1,000-mg doses (group A, $n = 15$) or four weekly 2,000-mg doses (group B, $n = 22$).[46]

ORR (primary endpoint) was 59% (47% group A, 68% group B). In 12 patients with baseline IgM $\geq$4 g/dL, ORR was 50% (17% group A, 83% group B). An improvement in anemia ($\geq$3 g/dL increase in hemoglobin) was seen in 58% of the 26 patients with baseline hemoglobin <11 g/dL (50% group A, 64% group B).

Ofatumumab was well tolerated in patients with WM. Infusion-related AEs occurred in 81% of patients (11% grade 3/4) and were manageable. Forty-one percent of patients had infections; most were grade 1/2. The incidence of IgM flare was low (5%). Further ofatumumab studies in WM are warranted, including combination strategies.

Clinical pharmacokinetics and pharmacodynamics of ofatumumab

Ofatumumab is cleared via two mechanisms: namely nonspecific clearance mechanisms as seen with other immunoglobulin G (IgG) molecules and target-mediated clearance via B cell binding.[9] The target-mediated clearance is highest at first infusion and is decreased at later doses. Statistically significant increases in half-life values and decreases in clearance values were found between the first and last infusions.[40,47] This is due to the rapid and sustained depletion of CD20$^+$ B cells after first infusion, leaving a reduced number of B cells available for antibody binding at subsequent infusions.[40] After repeated ofatumumab administration resulting in B cell depletion, clearance and volume of distribution

values were low and half-life values were long for ofatumumab, similar to values seen with other mAbs.[40,47]

The contribution of target-mediated clearance to the overall clearance of ofatumumab differs between diseases, with a greater effect of target-mediated clearance early in treatment of CLL than in FL. For example, the median overall clearance in patients with FL in study Hx-CD20-001 at doses of 300 to 1,000 mg at first infusion was 27 mL/h[48] but was 65 mL/h in patients with CLL who received 500 mg in study Hx-CD20-402;[47] median half-life values were 5.1 days in FL[48] and 1.3 days in CLL at first infusion.[47] At the fourth weekly infusion in these two studies, median clearance and half-life values were 9.5 mL/h and 17.1 days in patients with FL at doses of 300 to 1,000 mg and 10 mL/h and 13.6 days in patients with CLL at 2,000 mg, showing greater similarity after repeated administration and B cell depletion.[40,47]

Examination of potential covariates affecting ofatumumab pharmacokinetics other than diagnosis found that measures of body size (e.g., weight, body surface area) and gender had statistically significant but not clinically meaningful effects for which no dose adjustment is necessary. Other factors such as age and creatinine clearance had no significant effect. In an interim analysis of data from 146 patients with refractory CLL in study Hx-CD20-406, baseline measures of disease burden were associated with ofatumumab pharmacokinetics.[49]

Associations between ofatumumab exposure variables (e.g., C_{max}, C_{trough}, AUC) and clinical outcomes measures (e.g., ORR, PFS) were explored via regression analyses in patients with CLL and FL receiving ofatumumab monotherapy.[40,41,47,49] In univariate analyses in the FL studies,[40,41] higher ofatumumab exposure was not associated with ORR except for AUC at infusion 8 in study Hx-CD20-405; higher ofatumumab C_{max} and C_{trough} values at infusions 4 and 8 and AUC values at infusion 8 were associated with longer PFS in study Hx-CD20-405.[41] In contrast, univariate analyses in CLL studies found associations of higher C_{max}, C_{trough}, and AUC values at infusions 1, 4, or 8 with ORR as well as with longer PFS.[47,49] A multivariate analysis of the interim results of study Hx-CD20-406 in refractory CLL found that ofatumumab exposure variables were not significantly associated with either ORR or PFS when baseline disease characteristics and other factors identified in univariate analyses were included.[49] This finding suggests that ofatumumab exposure variables are not independent predictors of clinical outcomes in patients with refractory CLL.

Discussion

The management of CLL has become more personalized in recent years, in part due to a better understanding of genetic profiles that predict patient outcomes as well as increased treatment options permitting modification if toxicity is observed. In addition, combination therapies utilizing agents with distinct functional properties have improved treatment outcomes. Ofatumumab is an effective agent for the treatment of patients with CLL refractory to fludarabine and alemtuzumab. It has received accelerated approval from the FDA and conditional authorization by the EMA for this indication. The recent clinical trials highlighted in this review suggest it may have clinical benefit in patients with untreated CLL as well as other B cell malignancies. Ofatumumab has also been studied in the treatment of patients with nonmalignant diseases, including rheumatoid arthritis and multiple sclerosis.[50–53]

Emerging clinical evidence suggests that ofatumumab provides clinical benefit in patients with CLL in the frontline setting when combined with chemotherapy. The findings from the BIFROST trial have warranted the initiation of two large phase 3 trials testing ofatumumab plus chemotherapy, specifically chlorambucil or FC, in either frontline (COMPLEMENT 1) or second-line (COMPLEMENT 2) setting.

Another active area of research for ofatumumab is the maintenance setting in patients with advanced CLL who responded to induction therapy (PROLONG) or in patients with bulky fludarabine-refractory CLL (study OMB114242).

Current NCCN guidelines support the use of ofatumumab as monotherapy for treatment of patients with relapsed/refractory CLL with or without 11q or 17p deletions.[1] Ongoing studies depicted in Table 1 will determine if ofatumumab is warranted in other settings, such as in combination with chemotherapy or for frontline therapy of patients with CLL.

The initial clinical evaluation of ofatumumab in B-NHL (FL, DLBCL, and WM) has been encouraging. On the basis of promising results of ofatumumab monotherapy in patients with FL, a head-to-head phase 3 trial (HOMER) of ofatumumab monotherapy versus rituximab monotherapy in patients with relapsed FL after rituximab-based therapy was initiated. Based upon the MUNIN trial, showing that O-CHOP is a highly active chemoimmunotherapy regimen in the frontline therapy of FL, additional combination regimens are under evaluation in patients with indolent B-NHL, including a phase 3 study of ofatumumab plus bendamustine (COMPLEMENT A + B).

Phase 2 data on ofatumumab combination therapy in patients with relapsed/refractory DLBCL were promising, and a larger randomized trial comparing ofatumumab plus chemotherapy with rituximab plus chemotherapy (ORCHARRD) is ongoing. Phase 2 data on ofatumumab in WM demonstrated activity in this disease with an acceptable toxicity profile, warranting additional studies in patients with WM.

In summary, ofatumumab is active against several CD20[+] B cell hematologic malignancies, both as monotherapy (as evidenced in CLL, FL, DLBCL, and WM) and in combination with chemotherapy (as shown in CLL, FL, and DLBCL).

Acknowledgments

The authors would like to thank Francesca Balordi, Ph.D., of Medicus International New York, who provided writing assistance with funding from Glaxo-SmithKline.

Conflicts of interest

I.V.G. and R.C.J. are employees of GlaxoSmithKline and own stock in GlaxoSmithKline.

References

1. NCCN. "NCCN Clinical Practice Guidelines in Oncology. NCCN Non-Hodgkin's lymphoma Guidelines Vers 2," NCCN. Available at: www.nccn.org/professionals/physician_gls/f_guidelines.asp. Accessed 22 March 2012.
2. SEER. "Stat Fact Sheets: Chronic Lymphocytic Leukemia," Surveillance Epidemiology and End Results. Available at: http://seer.cancer.gov/statfacts/html/clyl.html. Accessed 22 March 2012.
3. SEER. "Fast Stats: Chronic Lymphocytic Leukemia Prevalence," Surveillance Epidemiology and End Results. Available at: http://seer.cancer.gov/faststats/selections.php?run−runit&output=2&data=5&statistic=9&race=1&sex=1&age=1&series=cancer&cancer=93#Output. Accessed 22 March 2012.
4. SEER. "Stat Fact Sheets: Non-Hodgkin Lymphoma," Surveillance Epidemiology and End Results. Available at:

http://seer.cancer.gov/statfacts/html/nhl.html#. Accessed 22 March 2012.

5. ACS. "Detailed Guide: 'What Is Non-Hodgkin Lymphoma?'," American Cancer Society. Available at: www.cancer.org/Cancer/Non-HodgkinLymphoma/ DetailedGuide/non-hodgkin-lymphoma-types-of-non-hodgkin-lymphoma. Accessed 22 March 2012.

6. Osterborg, A. 2010. Ofatumumab, a human anti-CD20 monoclonal antibody. *Expert. Opin. Biol. Ther.* **10:** 439–449.

7. NCCN. "NCCN Clinical Practice Guidelines in Oncology. NCCN Waldenstrom's macroglobulinemia/lymphoplasmacytic lymphoma Guidelines Vers 1," NCCN. Available at: www.nccn.org/professionals/physician_gls/f_guidelines.asp. Accessed 22 March 2012.

8. Genentech. "Rituxan (rituximab) prescribing information." Available at: www.gene.com/gene/products/information/pdf/rituxan-prescribing.pdf. Accessed 25 February 2012.

9. GlaxoSmithKline. "Arzerra (ofatumumab) prescribing information." Available at: www.gsksource.com/gskprm/htdocs/documents/ARZERRA.PDF. Accessed 25 February 2012.

10. GlaxoSmithKline. "Bexxar (tositumomab and iodine I 131 tositumomab) prescribing information." Available at: http://us.gsk.com/products/assets/us_bexxar.pdf. Accessed 4 April 2012.

11. Spectrum Pharmaceuticals Inc. "Zevalin (ibritumomab tiuxetan) prescribing information." Available at: www.zevalin.com/wp-content/uploads/2012/03/Zevalin_Package_Insert.pdf. Accessed 4 April 2012.

12. Genzyme. "Campath (alemtuzumab) prescribing information." Available at: www.campath.com/pdfs/2009-08-Campath%20US%20PI.pdf. Accessed 25 February 2012.

13. Cheson, B.D. 2010. Ofatumumab, a novel anti-CD20 monoclonal antibody for the treatment of B-cell malignancies. *J. Clin. Oncol.* **28:** 3525–3530.

14. Teeling, J.L. *et al.* 2006. The biological activity of human CD20 monoclonal antibodies is linked to unique epitopes on CD20. *J. Immunol.* **177:** 362–371.

15. Teeling, J.L. *et al.* 2004. Characterization of new human CD20 monoclonal antibodies with potent cytolytic activity against non-Hodgkin lymphomas. *Blood* **104:** 1793–1800.

16. Pawluczkowycz, A.W. *et al.* 2009. Binding of submaximal C1q promotes complement-dependent cytotoxicity (CDC) of B cells opsonized with anti-CD20 mAbs ofatumumab (OFA) or rituximab (RTX): considerably higher levels of CDC are induced by OFA than by RTX. *J. Immunol.* **183:** 749–758.

17. 2010. Ofatumumab (Arzerra) for CLL. *Med. Lett. Drugs Ther.* **52:** 51–52.

18. Bello, C., M. Veliz & J. Pinilla-Ibarz. 2011. Ofatumumab in the treatment of low-grade non-Hodgkin's lymphomas and chronic lymphocytic leukemia. *Expert Rev. Clin. Immunol.* **7:** 295–300.

19. Czuczman, M.S. & S.A. Gregory. 2010. The future of CD20 monoclonal antibody therapy in B-cell malignancies. *Leuk. Lymphoma* **51:** 983–994.

20. Nabhan, C. & N.E. Kay. 2011. The emerging role of ofatumumab in the treatment of chronic lymphocytic leukemia. *Clin. Med. Insights* **5:** 45–53.

21. Nightingale, G. 2011. Ofatumumab: a novel anti-CD20 monoclonal antibody for treatment of refractory chronic lymphocytic leukemia. *Ann. Pharmacother.* **45:** 1248–1255.

22. O'Brien, S. & A. Osterborg. 2010. Ofatumumab: a new CD20 monoclonal antibody therapy for B-cell chronic lymphocytic leukemia. *Clin. Lymphoma Myeloma Leuk.* **10:** 361–368.

23. Reagan, J.L. & J.J. Castillo. 2011. Ofatumumab for newly diagnosed and relapsed/refractory chronic lymphocytic leukemia. *Expert Rev. Anticancer Ther.* **11:** 151–160.

24. Robak, T. & E. Robak. 2011. New anti-CD20 monoclonal antibodies for the treatment of B-cell lymphoid malignancies. *BioDrugs* **25:** 13–25.

25. Sanford, M. & P.L. McCormack. 2010. Ofatumumab. *Drugs* **70:** 1013–1019.

26. Tsimberidou, A.M. 2010. Ofatumumab in the treatment of chronic lymphocytic leukemia. *Drugs Today (Barc)* **46:** 451–461.

27. Zhang, B. 2009. Ofatumumab. *mAbs* **1:** 326–331.

28. Coiffier, B. *et al.* 2008. Safety and efficacy of ofatumumab, a fully human monoclonal anti-CD20 antibody, in patients with relapsed or refractory B-cell chronic lymphocytic leukemia: a phase 1–2 study. *Blood* **111:** 1094–1100.

29. Wierda, W.G. *et al.* 2010. Ofatumumab as single-agent CD20 immunotherapy in fludarabine-refractory chronic lymphocytic leukemia. *J. Clin. Oncol.* **28:** 1749–1755.

30. Wierda, W.G. *et al.* 2010. Final analysis from the international trial of single-agent ofatumumab in patients with fludarabine-refractory chronic lymphocytic leukemia. Presented at the 52nd Annual Meeting of the American Society of Hematology, Orlando. *Blood* **116**. Abstract 921 (oral presentation).

31. O'Brien, S.M. *et al.* 2003. Alemtuzumab as treatment for residual disease after chemotherapy in patients with chronic lymphocytic leukemia. *Cancer* **98:** 2657–2663.

32. Keating, M.J. *et al.* 2002. Therapeutic role of alemtuzumab (Campath-1H) in patients who have failed fludarabine: results of a large international study. *Blood* **99:** 3554–3561.

33. Wierda, W.G. *et al.* 2011. Ofatumumab is active in patients with fludarabine-refractory CLL irrespective of prior rituximab: results from the phase 2 international study. *Blood* **118:** 5126–5129.

34. GlaxoSmithKline. "GSK and Genmab receive accelerated approval for Arzerra™," news release, April 19, 2010, October 26, 2009. Available at: www.gsk.com/media/pressreleases/2009/2009_us_pressrelease_10077.htm. Accessed 5 April 2012.

35. GlaxoSmithKline. "GlaxoSmithKline receives conditional marketing authorization in the EU for Arzerra® (ofatumumab)," news release, April 19, 2010. Available at: www.gsk.com/media/pressreleases/2010/2010_pressrelease_10038.htm. Accessed 5 April 2012.

36. Wierda, W.G. *et al.* 2011. Chemoimmunotherapy with O-FC in previously untreated patients with chronic lymphocytic leukemia. *Blood* **117:** 6450–6458.

37. Hallek, M. *et al.* 2010. Addition of rituximab to fludarabine and cyclophosphamide in patients with chronic lymphocytic leukaemia: a randomised, open-label, phase 3 trial. *Lancet* **376:** 1164–1174.

38. Keating, M.J. *et al*. 2005. Early results of a chemoim-munotherapy regimen of fludarabine, cyclophosphamide, and rituximab as initial therapy for chronic lymphocytic leukemia. *J. Clin. Oncol.* **23:** 4079–4088.

39. Tam, C.S. *et al*. 2008. Long-term results of the fludarabine, cyclophosphamide, and rituximab regimen as initial therapy of chronic lymphocytic leukemia. *Blood* **112:** 975–980.

40. Hagenbeek, A. *et al*. 2008. First clinical use of ofatumumab, a novel fully human anti-CD20 monoclonal antibody in relapsed or refractory follicular lymphoma: results of a phase 1/2 trial. *Blood* **111:** 5486–5495.

41. Czuczman, M.S. *et al*. 2012 Ofatumumab monotherapy in rituximab-refractory follicular lymphoma: results from a multicenter study. *Blood* **119:** 3698–3704.

42. Czuczman, M.S. *et al*. 2012. Chemoimmunotherapy with ofatumumab in combination with CHOP in previously untreated follicular lymphoma. *Br. J. Haematol.* **157:** 438–445.

43. Coiffier, B. *et al*. 2010. Ofatumumab monotherapy for treatment of patients with relapsed/progressive diffuse large B-cell lymphoma: results from a multicenter phase II study. Presented at the 52nd Annual Meeting of the American Society of Hematology, Orlando. *Blood* **116**. Abstract 3955 (poster presentation).

44. Matasar, M.J. *et al*. 2011. A phase II study of ofatumumab in combination with ICE or DHAP chemotherapy in relapsed or refractory aggressive B-cell lymphoma prior to autologous stem cell transplantation (ASCT). Presented at the 53rd Annual Meeting of the American Society of Hematology, San Diego. *Blood* **118**. Abstract 957 (oral presentation).

45. Gisselbrecht, C. *et al*. 2010. Salvage regimens with autologous transplantation for relapsed large B-cell lymphoma in the rituximab era. *J. Clin. Oncol.* **28:** 4184–4190.

46. Furman, R.R. *et al*. 2011. A phase II trial of ofatumumab in subjects with Waldenstrom's macroglobulinemia. Presented at the 53rd Annual Meeting of the American Society of Hematology, San Diego. *Blood* **118**. Abstract 3701 (poster presentation).

47. Coiffier, B. *et al*. 2010. Pharmacokinetics and pharmacokinetic/pharmacodynamic associations of ofatumumab, a human monoclonal CD20 antibody, in patients with relapsed or refractory chronic lymphocytic leukaemia: a phase 1–2 study. *Br. J. Haematol.* **150:** 58–71.

48. GlaxoSmithKline. Data on file.

49. Österborg, A. *et al*. 2009. Correlation between serum ofatumumab concentrations, baseline patient characteristics and clinical outcomes in patients with fludarabine-refractory chronic lymphocytic leukemia (CLL) treated with single-agent ofatumumab. Presented at the 51st Annual Meeting of the American Society of Hematology, New Orleans. *Blood* **114**. Abstract 3433 (poster presentation).

50. Ostergaard, M. *et al*. 2010. Ofatumumab, a human anti-CD20 monoclonal antibody, for treatment of rheumatoid arthritis with an inadequate response to one or more disease-modifying antirheumatic drugs: results of a randomized, double-blind, placebo-controlled, phase I/II study. *Arthritis Rheum.* **62:** 2227–2238.

51. GlaxoSmithKline. "Investigating clinical efficacy of ofatumumab in adult rheumatoid arthritis (RA) patients who had an inadequate response to TNF-α antagonist." Available at: www.clinicaltrials.gov/ct2/results?term=NCT00603525. Accessed 22 March 2012.

52. GlaxoSmithKline. "Investigating clinical efficacy of ofatumumab in adult rheumatoid arthritis (RA) patients who had an inadequate response to methotrexate therapy." Available at: www.clinicaltrials.gov/ct2/results?term=NCT00611455. Accessed 22 March 2012.

53. GlaxoSmithKline. "Ofatumumab dose-finding in relapsing remitting multiple sclerosis patients." Available at: www.clinicaltrials.gov/ct2/results?term=NCT00640328. Accessed 22 March 2012.

54. GlaxoSmithKline. "A single-arm, international, multicenter trial investigating the efficacy and safety of ofatumumab retreatment and maintenance in CLL patients who progressed following response or stable disease after ofatumumab treatment in Hx-CD20-406." Available at: www.clinicaltrials.gov/ct2/show/NCT00802737?term–NCT 00802737&rank=1. Accessed 22 March 2012.

55. GlaxoSmithKline. "A phase III, open label, randomized, multicenter trial of ofatumumab maintenance treatment versus no further treatment in subjects with relapsed chronic lymphocytic leukemia (CLL) who have responded to induction therapy (PROLONG)." Available at: www.clinicaltrials.gov/ct2/show/NCT01039376? term=NCT01039376&rank=1. Accessed 5 April 2012.

56. GlaxoSmithKline. "An open label, multicenter study investigating the safety and efficacy of ofatumumab therapy versus physicians' choice in patients with bulky fludarabine-refractory chronic lymphocytic leukaemia (CLL)." Available at: www.clinicaltrials.gov/ct2/show/NCT01313689? term=NCT01313689&rank=1. Accessed 22 March 2012.

57. GlaxoSmithKline. "A phase II, multi-centre study investigating the safety and efficacy of ofatumumab and ben damustine combination in patients with untreated or relapsed chronic lymphocytic leukaemia (CLL)." Available at: www.clinicaltrials.gov/ct2/show/NCT01520922?term= NCT01520922&rank=1. Accessed 22 March 2012.

58. GlaxoSmithKline. "A phase III, open label, randomized, multicenter trial of ofatumumab added to chlorambucil versus chlorambucil monotherapy in previously untreated patients with chronic lymphocytic leukemia (COMPLEMENT 1)." Available at: www.clinicaltrials.gov/ct2/show/ NCT00748189?term=NCT00748189&rank=1. Accessed 22 March 2012.

59. GlaxoSmithKline. "A phase III, open label, randomized trial of ofatumumab added to fludarabine-cyclophosphamide vs. fludarabine-cyclophosphamide combination in subjects with relapsed chronic lymphocytic leukemia (COMPLEMENT 2)." Available at: www.clinicaltrials.gov/ ct2/show/NCT00824265?term=NCT00824265&rank=1. Accessed 22 March 2012.

60. GlaxoSmithKline. "Phase III randomized, open label study of single agent ofatumumab versus single agent rituximab in follicular lymphoma relapsed after rituximab-containing therapy (HOMER)." Available at: www.clinicaltrials.gov/ ct2/show/NCT01200589?term=NCT01200589&rank=1. Accessed 22 March 2012.

61. GlaxoSmithKline. "A randomized, open label study of ofatumumab and bendamustine combination therapy

compared with bendamustine monotherapy in indolent B-cell non-Hodgkin's lymphoma unresponsive to rituximab or a rituximab-containing regimen during or within six months of treatment (COMPLEMENT A+B)." Available at: www.clinicaltrials.gov/ct2/show/NCT01077518?term=NCT01077518&rank=1. Accessed 22 March 2012.

62. GlaxoSmithKline. "Ofatumumab versus rituximab salvage chemoimmunotherapy followed by autologous stem cell transplant in relapsed or refractory diffuse large B cell lymphoma (ORCHARRD)." Available at: www.clinicaltrials.gov/ct2/show/NCT01014208?term=NCT01014208&rank=1. Accessed 22 March 2012.